Recipes for

IBS

IRRITABLE BOWEL SYNDROME

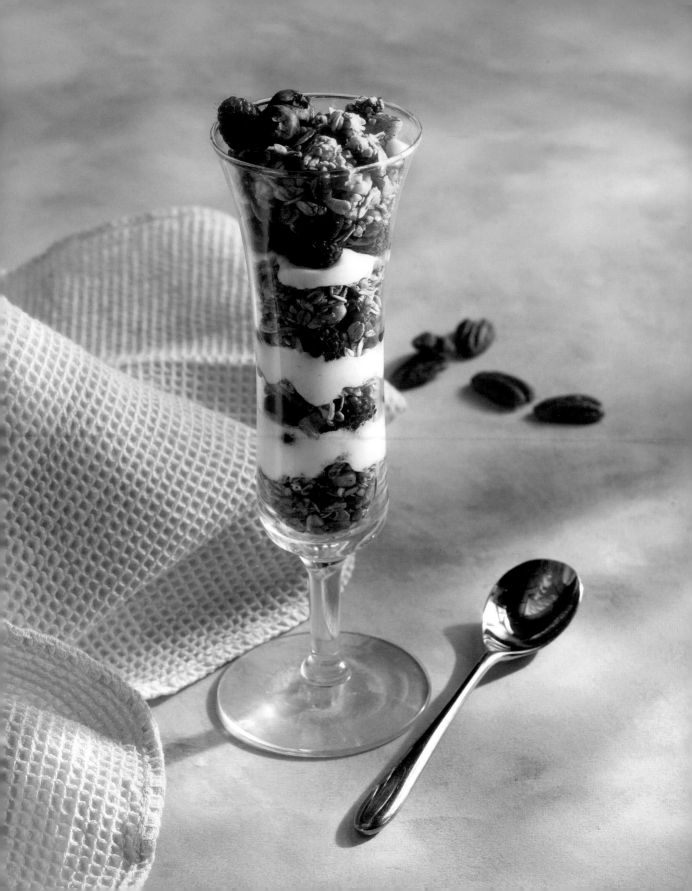

Recipes for

IBS

IRRITABLE BOWEL SYNDROME

Great Tasting Recipes and Tips Customized for *Your* Symptoms

Ashley Koff, R.D.

Foreword by Sonia Friedman, M.D.

First published in the USA in 2007 by
Fair Winds Press, a member of
Quayside Publishing Group
33 Commercial Street
Gloucester, MA 01930

11 10 09 08 07   1 2 3 4 5

ISBN-13: 978-1-59233-230-4
ISBN-10: 1-59233-230-7

Library of Congress Cataloging-in-Publication Data available

Cover design by Howard Grossman/12e Design
Book design by Yee Design
Photography by Steve Galvin

Printed and bound in China

This book is not intended to replace the services of a physician. Any application of the recommendations set forth in the following pages is at the reader's discretion. The reader should consult with his or her own physician or specialist concerning the recommendations in this book.

Contents

Foreword

As long ago as 1849, W. Cumming, a physician, wrote, "The bowels are at one time constipated, at another lax, in the same person. How the disease has two such different symptoms I do not profess to explain...." This description of irritable bowel syndrome (IBS) is still accurate today. In fact, irritable bowel syndrome is much more prevalent than most people realize. It affects 10 to 20 percent of the adult American population and is the most common diagnosis made by gastroenterologists. The symptoms of IBS are chronic or recurrent lower abdominal pain or discomfort, altered bowel function, and bloating. Patients usually have urgency, altered stool consistency, altered stool frequency, and/or incomplete evacuation. IBS can cause great discomfort, sometimes on and off and other times continuously, for many decades in a person's life. The estimated total healthcare costs associated with IBS are about $21 billion dollars a year. The direct costs in diagnostic tests, physician and emergency room visits, hospitalizations, and medications are $1 billion. The indirect costs in reduced work productivity, absenteeism, and travel to consultations are about $20 billion.[1] Of course these estimates leave out the intangible costs of human suffering and impaired quality of life.

In the United States, about two-thirds of patients who suffer from IBS are women. This may be due to the fact that women more readily report their symptoms of abdominal pain, gas, bloating, and altered bowel movements. It may also be due to hormonal differences between men and women that may affect gut function and alter perception of pain due to abdominal distention. IBS primarily affects people in the prime of their lives—between the ages of twenty and forty. Patient surveys from both the United States and the United Kingdom report an average disease duration of eleven years with one-third of patients having symptoms for much longer.[2,3] For many patients, symptoms occur frequently and significantly impair emotional, physical, and social well-being. Almost three-fourths of patients report symptoms more than once a week and about half report daily symptoms. In a telephone survey of female IBS sufferers in the United States, almost 40 percent reported pain and discomfort as intolerable without relief. Women with IBS reported 71 percent more abdominal surgeries than women without IBS. The rates of gallbladder operations, hysterectomies, and appendectomies were twice as high or higher among women with IBS. Twenty-five percent had been hospitalized overnight due to symptoms. Seventy-eight percent of women had limits on what they ate, 43 percent had limits on sports and recreational activity, 43 percent on social activity, 40 percent on vacation and travel, and 28 percent on sexual activity. Two-thirds of women were concerned about restroom availability wherever they went, one-third avoided group meetings, and 25 percent got up earlier for work.

Even more frustrating was that only 39 percent of women were diagnosed with IBS by the first physician they saw. Three percent saw eight or more physicians before getting a diagnosis. Time from onset to diagnosis took an average of three years, and patients saw an average of three physicians before getting a diagnosis.

IBS also affects productivity at work. IBS sufferers are absent an average of thirteen days per year due to symptoms, versus non-IBS sufferers who are absent an average of five days per year.[4] In a recent study that compared quality of life among patients with IBS, migraine, asthma, esophageal reflux, and subjects in the general U.S. population, IBS patients had a significantly worse quality of life on all levels. IBS patients had decreased physical functioning, increased body pain, worse general health, vitality, social functioning, emotional, and mental health.[5]

What Exactly Is IBS?

What causes the increased gas, bloating, pain, and altered bowel movements? Historical terms describing IBS include spastic colon, irritable colon, unstable colon, nervous colon, and mucous colitis. In 1966 a physician, CJ DeLor, coined the name irritable bowel syndrome, which exists today. These historical names are interesting because they describe the endpoint of bowel pain and spasm without describing the "why" and "how." In the 1960s and 70s, IBS was thought to be due to abnormal motility or movement of the small intestine and colon. In the 1980s and 90s it was thought to be due to an increased perception of pain to abdominal distention. To test this theory, investigators inflated a small balloon in the sigmoid colon of several IBS patients and non-IBS patients. Even with the same amount of air, IBS patients felt much more pain than non-IBS patients. Investigators then immersed the hands of IBS and non-IBS patients in ice water. The perception of pain was exactly the same. This experiment tells us that the heightened pain sensation is specific to the gut in IBS patients.[6]

More recently, the brains of IBS patients have been studied by a test called a functional MRI. The special MRI locates the area of the brain that is activated by distending the sigmoid colon with air. In fact, different areas in IBS patients and non-patients will "light up" on the MRI. This tells us that the brains of IBS and non-IBS patients respond differently to pain. In addition, there are many connections between the brain, spinal cord, and the gut. The gut will literally tell the brain how to respond when the colon is distended, and this response will be different in patients with IBS.[7,8]

In addition, the gut has a brain of its own. Amazingly, the gut contains 90 percent as many neurons, or nerve cells, as there are in the brain. The main chemical that controls pain sensation, gut motility, and secretion of water in the intestine is serotonin. Ninety-five percent of the nerve cells that contain serotonin are in the gut. Serotonin controls gut sensitivity and helps control consistency of stool, preventing it from becoming too hard or too soft and causing constipation or diarrhea. Serotonin is also present in the brain and is involved in modulating the brain's response to pain. IBS patients may have different levels of serotonin in the gut and most likely in the brain. What this means is that IBS patients should know that their symptoms are real. They are not "crazy" or too "stressed-out." Although stress, psychological state, coping skills, and social support can play a role in IBS, they are not the cause. What modern research will likely show is that it all comes down to altered levels of serotonin in the brain and in the gut.[9,10]

Even more interesting is that there is some evidence of a link between inappropriate inflammation and IBS. IBS patients may have increased inflammation in the gut on a microscopic level and increased inflammatory factors in the bloodstream. This increased inflammation may lead to an altered level of serotonin in the gut and may play a role in causing IBS.[11]

How Is IBS Diagnosed?

There are specific medical criteria, called the ROME II criteria, which aid in the diagnosis of IBS. Patients should have for at least twelve weeks, which need not be consecutive, in the preceding twelve months, abdominal discomfort or pain that has two of the following three features: relieved with defecation, onset associated with a change in stool frequency, and onset associated with a change in form (appearance) of stool.[12] It is uncommon for the first IBS symptoms to present after age forty. Physicians ask patients about "red flag" symptoms, including rectal bleeding, weight loss greater than ten pounds, family history of colon cancer, recurring fevers, low blood count, and nighttime diarrhea. As part of the initial evaluation, a blood count and thyroid test should be drawn and an abdominal and rectal exam performed. Patients are questioned about any history in the immediate family of Crohn's disease, ulcerative colitis, or colon cancer. Physicians ask patients about milk or wheat intolerance as well and might do a blood test for celiac sprue or a breath test for milk intolerance. For a patient over forty years old first presenting with symptoms of IBS, or a patient with blood on a rectal exam, a colonoscopy is recommended. About 30 to

40 percent of patients with severe IBS have a history of physical or sexual abuse, and physicians should always ask about this. For these patients, psychotherapy is helpful and may alleviate bowel symptoms.

Treating IBS

The current management of IBS has multiple components. Perhaps the two most important parts of the treatment plan are education and reassurance. The more time physicians take to talk to their patients, the more happy and self-sufficient patients are in general. Dietary modification is an important part of IBS therapy and this cookbook, written by Ashley Koff, R.D., a dietitian specializing in digestive function and integrative medicine, who has treated hundreds of IBS patients, is an essential guide to nutritional therapy for IBS management and treatment. Fiber found in whole grains, fruits, nuts, seeds, and vegetables and also in the form of fiber supplements containing psyllium (Metamucil), guar gum (Benefiber), calcium polycarbofil (Fibercon), and methylcellulose (Citrucel) help to regulate bowel movements and improve stool consistency. Additionally, medications are available to help treat IBS symptoms. One of the most important things for patients to remember is that they must set realistic treatment goals. With proper medical, dietary, and sometimes psychological therapy, patients can achieve a significant improvement in quality of life.

Medical Treatment for IBS

Medical treatment for IBS differs depending upon the severity of the disease. For mild to moderate IBS, it is helpful to treat the dominant symptoms of pain, bloating, and/or altered bowel motility.

For abdominal pain, antispasmotic agents are helpful. They relax the smooth muscle of the gut. They include dicyclomine hydrochloride (Bentyl), hyoscyamine sulfate (Anaspaz, Levsin), atropine (Lomotil), scopolamine and phenobarbital (Donnatal), and clidinium bromide with chlordiazepoxide (Librax). These medicines are usually given before meals to inhibit abdominal pain and immediate, uncontrolled bowel movements.

Tricyclic antidepressants such as amitriptyline hydrochloride (Elavil) and nortriptyline hydrochloride (Pamelor), prescribed at low doses, are beneficial in patients with and without diagnosed depression and anxiety as their benefit is more for pain reduction than depression. Side effects of both antispasmodics and tricyclics include dry mouth, dry eyes, and fatigue.

More recently, citalopram hydrobromide (Celexa) has been tested in patients with IBS. One study found that this selective serotonin reuptake inhibitor, which is commonly used for depression, was effective in patients with IBS. Citalopram significantly improved symptoms of abdominal pain and bloating and improved quality of life and overall well-being.[13] Fluoxitine hydrochloride (Prozac), another serotonin reuptake inhibitor commonly used for depression, is also effective in treating IBS. In a study last year in patients with constipation-predominant IBS, fluoxetine decreased abdominal discomfort and bloating and increased bowel movements.[14]

For patients whose main trouble is altered bowel movements, and for whom dietary and lifestyle modifications prove ineffective, there are medications that can help. For those with diarrhea, loperamide hydrochloride (Imodium) can help slow down bowel movements. Cholestyramine (Questran) binds bile acids in the small intestine and helps slow down diarrhea. For those with constipation, the first steps should be to increase dietary fiber through food choices, ensure adequate hydration and encourage motility with activity. Next, consider fiber supplementation. If these fail, there are different types of laxatives that can help. These include senna and bisacodyl (Dulcolax). While senna and bisacodyl can be very helpful in the short term, they should not be used over months to years because they might cause dilation of the bowel and may no longer be effective. Laxatives that can be used safely on a daily basis include polyethylene glycol (MiraLax) and lactulose (Cephulac). Polyethylene glycol comes in a powder form and can be mixed in water, decaffeinated tea, or diluted juice. Lactulose comes in a syrup form and should be consumed with a minimum of eight ounces of water. (It's ok to add a splash of juice or lemon.) All of these "osmotic" laxatives cause retention of water in the stool and help make bowel movements softer and more frequent. The side effects of osmotic laxatives include occasional increased gas and abdominal cramping. Potential side effects should not be discouraging, however. What works for one patient may not work for another.

Enemas and Suppositories

Many patients ask about enemas and suppositories. For patients who need them for intractable constipation, the vast majority will use only them occasionally. The safest suppository to use is a glycerin suppository since it is not a stimulant laxative and has no lasting ill effects on the gut. It is the rare individual who needs these on a daily basis and if this occurs it should be under the guidance of a physician.

New Medications to Treat IBS

The newer medications for IBS do not just treat the symptoms; they attempt to treat the cause. Alosetron hydrochloride (Lotronex) is a medication for women with severe diarrhea-predominant IBS. It blocks serotonin receptors in the gut and reduces gut motility, pain sensation, and intestinal secretions. Many patients may have heard the bad press about Lotronex. Initially, the drug was launched in February

2000. It was withdrawn from the market November 2000 due to side effects of constipation and ischemic colitis or lack of blood flow to the colon. There were three deaths and seventy-seven hospitalizations due to these diagnoses. The drug was approved for reintroduction in June 2002. Physicians who prescribe it must be enrolled in a special program, and the patient and physician must sign a consent agreement. In reality, if alosetron is prescribed correctly, and if the treating physician manages the patient closely, this drug can be extremely helpful and safe. A handful of patients are severely debilitated by abdominal pain and diarrhea, and their lives can be significantly improved with alosetron. Many of these patients would otherwise be on narcotics or sedatives.

Tegaserod maleate (Zelnorm) is the opposite of alosetron. It stimulates serotonin receptors in the gut, increases fluid secretions and gut motility, and decreases pain sensation in the gut. It normalizes bowel function and relieves abdominal pain and discomfort in women with constipation-predominant IBS. It is approved for both men and women with chronic constipation. Medical studies have documented increased bowel movements, decreased straining, decreased bloating, and increased quality of life with tegaserod.[15] The initial side effects of tegaserod include diarrhea and headache, but these usually get better. It is a very useful drug for IBS patients whose symptoms haven't improved with or who have been intolerant of fiber and/or laxative therapy.

A Review of IBS

There is no one right way to treat IBS, and treatment is often a trial and error process. The most important thing in treating IBS is the therapeutic relationship between the patient and the physician. Patients should report their symptoms honestly and thoroughly (don't be afraid to be graphic), and physicians should appreciate any awkwardness and/or frustration such reporting presents. This way, each interaction can be viewed as a continued effort to identify a successful treatment for that patient.

A review of IBS would not be complete without a discussion of the psychological treatments. Patients with severe IBS frequently have a history of depression or physical or sexual abuse. Programs that have shown to help in moderate to severe IBS include psychotherapy, stress management/relaxation therapy, biofeedback, and hypnotherapy.

Perhaps one of the most interesting potential therapies in IBS is probiotics. These are natural beneficial bacteria that are normally present in a healthy digestive tract. The concept is that they will replenish the good (sometimes called "friendly") bacteria in the gastrointestinal tract. In a recent medical study, Bifidobacterium infantis 35624 was shown to alleviate abdominal pain and bloating and bowel movement difficulty.[16] Another probiotic, which contains eight different strains of bacteria including lactobacillus and bifidobacteria, alleviated flatulence and slowed down stools in IBS patients. More studies are needed to support probiotics as a primary therapy, and since they are non-prescription, cost can be a factor as well.

Along the same line of using probiotics, an antibiotic, rifaximin (Xifaxan), has been shown to help symptoms of bloating and flatulence. This is a special type of antibiotic because it is not absorbed in the bloodstream; it treats bad bacteria only in the gastrointestinal tract. Thus, the side effects should be minimal and the medicine safe. The first U.S. trial of this medication in IBS was in February 2006, and more trials need to be done.

Complementary therapies for IBS that may help alleviate symptoms—according to individual testimony or practitioners' anecdotal reports—include acupuncture, meditation, nutritional supplements, hot baths, abdominal massage, and herbalist treatments.

Diagnosing IBS should include assessments for food intolerances and allergies. It is important to make sure you do not have celiac disease, which is an immune reaction of the gut to gluten and can simulate symptoms of IBS. Celiac disease occurs in about 1 in 250 people in the United States and testing can be done with a simple blood test. Patients with celiac disease must be on a strict gluten-free diet. Lactose intolerance is very common and can also cause the same symptoms as IBS. It is seen in 7 to 20 percent of Caucasians, as high as 80 to 95 percent of Native Americans, 65 to 75 percent of Africans and African Americans, and 50 percent of Hispanics. The prevalence is greater than 90 percent in some populations in Eastern Asia. It is ruled out by a simple breath test. For people who are lactose intolerant, lactase preparations such as Lactaid, Lactrase, and Dairy Ease may help, but many patients will still have symptoms and will have to avoid all lactose-containing food products. Food allergies are much rarer but do occur and an allergy specialist can do skin testing for these. Patients with food allergies will usually have a skin rash in addition to gastrointestinal symptoms.

What Should and Shouldn't I Eat?

Probably the most common question IBS patients ask me is, "What should and shouldn't I eat?" Often patients get widely different and confusing advice from friends and dietitians. Since each patient is different, IBS patients should receive individualized counseling from only registered dietitians specializing in digestive disorders for guidance in developing a personalized nutrition plan. In this cookbook, Ashley Koff, R.D., offers an insightful and extremely useful guide to nutrition therapy for all types of IBS. She provides recipes and numerous dietary and lifestyle modifications based on her own vast experience with IBS patients. Her recipes are organized and color-coded by IBS symptoms and were created to help patients with all types of IBS enjoy their food without regrets. These recipes will be an asset to IBS patients and a perfect complement to traditional medical therapy.

Sonia Friedman, M.D.
Assistant Professor of Medicine
Harvard Medical School
Associate Physician
Brigham and Women's Hospital

CHAPTER 1

The Recipe for IBS Treatment

As Dr. Friedman stated in her foreword, the most popular question IBS patients ask is, "What should or shouldn't I eat?" Thus, a cookbook for IBS patients makes perfect sense. But is "what should or shouldn't I eat" the whole issue? Or should we ask, *"How* can I treat my IBS?" *Recipes for IBS* answers this question by providing information about good choices and how to implement them for a healthy eating and lifestyle plan—the recipe for IBS treatment.

Just as a recipe is made up of several ingredients that combine to make a delicious dish, *your* recipe for IBS treatment will be made up of several ingredients that combine for the delicious result of good health, beginning with reduced IBS symptoms. This cookbook goes beyond the healing properties and palate-pleasing experiences of individual recipes to present you with the knowledge and skills that are critical to the successful treatment of IBS. Read on to experience how good overcoming IBS can taste and feel!

INGREDIENT 1

Quality Basics

The first "ingredient" in our recipe for IBS treatment is using quality basics. The quality of the basic ingredients in a recipe can do as much, if not more, to determine the final outcome of the dish. In this book, quality basics means starting with the best choices, which are those that prioritize both the treatment of IBS and the improvement of overall health.

Quality: It's *Your* Choice

IBS nutrition tends to be, well, just basic nutrition. One of the most disconcerting complaints I hear from IBS patients is that their symptoms prevent them from a healthy lifestyle, caused by food restrictions, activity limitations, or both. For example, some people use their fear of triggering IBS symptoms to justify lower-quality dietary choices *because they are easier on my system.* These people might avoid fruits, vegetables, and beans; rely on less nutrient-dense foods from these categories; emphasize calorie-dense, nutrient-poor *food products*, which are processed versions of whole foods that bear minimal nutrition resemblance to their whole food relatives.

While the error of such choices frustrates me, the blame does not lie exclusively with the IBS patient. Healthcare practitioners—including doctors, nurses, *and* dietitians—share at least an equal part of the blame. Patient education efforts, typically in the form of handouts, may actually endorse suboptimal health choices. Handouts listing "foods to avoid," which are also called "trigger foods" for their potential to trigger IBS symptoms, typically list together, without distinction, highly nutritious foods as well as less quality foods and non-nutritive food products. These handouts either lack replacement suggestions altogether, offer replacement suggestions that are lower-quality than the original food, or lack suggestions *of equal quality* for the high-quality choices on the list. Because guidelines emphasizing food replacements of equal nutritional quality are absent, patients are on their own to identify appropriate food choices. Thus, their food choices tend to be those that they sense will be "easier on my system." And finally, handouts rarely distinguish triggers for different symptoms—such as constipation, diarrhea, and indigestion—so patients often avoid a food or group of foods that aren't really a likely trigger for their symptoms, but could actually contain health benefits, including symptom relief.

Today, there is an impressive amount of nutrition information available. Fortunately, there is growing consensus that it is the *type* of foods, the *quality* that one consumes, that promote health. Quality choices, paired with appropriate quantity, encourage the body's natural ability to function optimally, prevent disease, and heal itself.

Quality is about making choices. What you choose *not* to eat is as important as what you choose *to* eat.

CHOOSE *TO* EAT AS OFTEN AS POSSIBLE	CHOOSE *NOT* TO EAT AS OFTEN AS POSSIBLE
Food—things that you would find in nature.	*Food products*—anything you couldn't make in your kitchen. I ask my youngest clients to tell me how they'd make Hot Cheetos or Froot Loops. Make it a policy to avoid all trans fats (partially hydrogenated oils) and high fructose corn syrup.
If there's a label, you should recognize the words listed on the ingredient label as foods or spices.	Labels with items you can't define.
Whole foods (in appropriate quantities) for their natural nutrient balance and satisfaction.	Pre-prepared meals, including bars and shakes when you can make your own. These meals may contain digestive irritants, and they may be deficient in good things such as fiber and excessive in others such as calories.
New foods daily and on a seasonal basis.	The same thing everyday. Your body *and* soul will get bored.
Fruits or vegetables in place of the juice. The skins, pulps, and cells are packed with nutrients. If you choose juice, make it yourself and keep your portions appropriate.	Fruit products (fruit leather, jellies, Jell-O, etc.) in place of eating whole fruit.
Include vegetable sources of protein more often as they provide fiber and other valuable nutrients for health. Try the more easily digestible options—such as mung, aduki beans, quinoa, buckwheat, and amaranth—at first.	Eat animal protein exclusively as a way to avoid carbs. Carbs are not the enemy; *quality* carbs in the right *quantity* are a valued part of a healthy nutrition plan.
Include vegetables at meals and snacks to help you feel full. Choose to explore different preparations, such as cooked, sautéed, in soups, and as a dipper.	*More* animal protein or fat to feel full. Too much of either at one time challenges your digestive system.
Meals full of natural color.	One-color or colorless meals. I challenge my youngest clients to make their plates a rainbow, and Froot Loops or Skittles don't count!
Fruits and vegetables with dark-colored flesh or leaves.	Vegetables without color (iceberg lettuce, white potato, etc.) exclusively.
Fresh and frozen fruits and vegetables much more often than canned or dried.	Fruits and vegetables that are sitting out for too long or packaged poorly.
Just take a taste of different dishes when dining out and, to be safe, order a basic side that you like and you know your system will tolerate.	The whole portion that's given to you at a restaurant. It's not just for calorie control. Also your digestive system functions best when it's not overwhelmed.
Grains in their whole form more often.	Refined grains (*white* bread, crackers, etc.) or flour-based (bread, pasta, crackers) carbohydrates at every meal. Explore root vegetables, legumes, etc.

CHOOSE *TO* EAT AS OFTEN AS POSSIBLE	CHOOSE *NOT* TO EAT AS OFTEN AS POSSIBLE
Wheat-free grains such as quinoa, amaranth, teff, buckwheat, oats, rice, and wild rice. They offer additional, valuable nutrients.	Wheat every time you want a grain.
Organic, locally grown, hormone-free, preservative-free foods when possible.	Chemicals. Or at least limit your intake of them.
Drink water, herbal teas, and healing tonics, which are nutrient-rich and calorie-appropriate.	Frequently drink nutrient poor, high-calorie, or artificially sweetened beverages.
Dishes that are inherently flavorful by cooking with spices and herbs.	Foods hidden beneath sauces of unknown origin or to heap on your own sauce after the food is prepared.
A snack *now* to prevent overeating or poor choices later.	Food just because it's around.

A word on *food* versus *food products*: Many food products today barely resemble their whole food relative. Routine consumption of processed foods cheats your body's digestive system, which is built to break down foods and to allocate nutrients according to need and priority. To eat or drink this way is like watching an exercise video from the couch. It may sound good and lounging on the couch for a day may even *feel* good, but in the long run you get flabby, crabby, and ultimately lose out. Routine consumption of processed foods makes our bodies lazy, and with laziness comes inefficiency and error. And, in this case, inefficiency and error can translate into disease.

A word on whole grains versus processed grains: think "Grain before flour, gives you more power"—digestive power that is. By preferentially consuming flour-based products (these include whole grain flour), over whole grains, we create lazy guts. Grains make our systems work the way they're meant to and that helps optimize body functions, such as metabolism, digestion, and circulation. Go for whole grains more often.

The Principles: Foods That Heal

The second "ingredient" in our recipe for IBS treatment is healing foods. Most people choose recipes based on their main ingredients. You might be attracted to how the ingredient tastes, its texture, its appearance, or a combination of these qualities. In this book, foods that heal are the main ingredients. And their most attractive qualities are their healing properties. As Hippocrates said, **"Let food be thy medicine, and let thy medicine be thy food."**

The following foods, herbs, and spices are especially beneficial for your digestive system. Foods not included on this list are still worthwhile unless noted in "the replacements" on page 19. Throughout this book, these ingredients are mixed and matched into delicious recipes so that every bite you take and sip you drink helps you to manage your symptoms and heal, as well as satiate and please. Because this is ultimately *your recipe,* I encourage you to return to this list to come up with your own recipe modifications.

A word of caution: While these foods contain healing properties, it's important to eat the ones that are best for you. Use the color code system (see page 37) in this book to find the right foods for your particular symptom. For example, sesame seed and spinach are great for constipation, but they're not advised for loose stools or diarrhea.

- **FRUITS AND VEGETABLES**: apples, avocados, bananas, beets, berries, carrots, dark leafy greens (beet, collards, kale, mustard, spinach, etc.), fennel, figs, kiwis, lemons, limes, mangoes, mushrooms, okra, olives, papayas, parsnips, persimmons, prunes, pumpkins, quinces, rutabagas, seaweeds, squashes, sweet potatoes or yams, and turnips

  Note that apples and prunes may be difficult to eat raw or with the skins on. Start by removing the skins or eating them baked or cooked and mashed.

  Only lemons and limes are listed as healing foods, as opposed to other citrus fruits, because lemons and limes are known as weak acids, while other citrus fruits are strongly acidic. Weak acids actually work to stimulate the release of bicarbonate in the small intestine, and in doing so encourage a more alkaline state in the lower digestive tract, which is positive.

  Leafy greens should have stems removed, and they are best cooked, such as steamed, sautéed, or added to soups.

  While starchy fruits and vegetables—such as bananas, beets, carrots, parsnips, pumpkin, rutabagas, squashes, sweet potatoes or yams, and turnips—aid the digestive system, eat them with attention to quantity and nutrient variety.

- **HERBS AND SPICES:** basil, caraway, carob, chamomile, chicory, cinnamon, citrus peel, cumin, dandelion, fennel, fenugreek, ginger, lavender, mint, parsley, saffron, and turmeric

- **NUTS AND SEEDS:** almonds, chia, flax, hemp, pine nuts, pistachio, pumpkin, sesame (black), sunflower, and walnuts

  Note: Store nuts and seeds in the refrigerator or freezer to prevent oxidation. Try their oils and butters (especially if the whole seed or nut bothers your system) and review the websites in the resource section for proper usage when cooking and storage.

- **GRAINS:** amaranth, barley, buckwheat (soba), corn meal (polenta), millet, quinoa, oat, rice, and teff

- **BRANS:** rice, oat, psyllium

- **LEGUMES:** adzuki beans, lentils, mung, and tempeh

- **ANIMAL PROTEINS:** sardines, wild cod and salmon, and hormone free, grass fed lean meats

  Note: Grass feeding encourages the production of a better ratio of fatty acids in the meat. The switch to *grain-fed* from *grass-fed* is something that is now identified in terms of decreasing the nutritive quality of our meats—also, grain-fed animals are more likely to need antibiotics, as the grains cause an accumulation of bacteria in the guts of cows and other animals that aren't meant to eat the grain feed.

INGREDIENT 3

The Supporting Cast: The Replacements

When you cook, you can prepare a recipe exactly as it was written or you can modify it based on your preference or need. But when you modify a recipe by taking out an ingredient, you must first assess the contributions of that ingredient to the recipe. Then you should choose another ingredient to replace that ingredient's contributions. For example, let's say a recipe calls for tomato as a garnish. If you need or want to avoid tomatoes, it is quite easy to replace the tomato; however, if the recipe is a tomato-rice soup, it's probably better to find a different recipe. For people with IBS, replacing ingredients that are gastric irritants with complementary ingredients reduces irritation, helps reduce other symptoms, and ultimately allows your body to concentrate on healing.

Some foods, beverages, and substances can be replaced relatively easily, whereas others require too much work to balance out their negative impact on the digestive system. Especially in the initial phases of dietary modifications, reducing quantity may be an effective first replacement, as well as changing preparation method, or employing food combining techniques. Sometimes people have a hard time finding a replacement for favorite foods. I often ask them to complete a food and mood journal or to tell me why they love a particular food. This helps them select an appropriate replacement.

The same food or beverage can be a favorite for many people, but *why* it's a favorite can differ for each person. Likewise, your favorite may satisfy different needs based on timing, mood, environment, and more. For example, several of my patients began our first session telling me they couldn't give up "my coffee." Yet, when I probed, I discovered that "my coffee" means something different to each of them. For one patient, coffee is physiological. She needs the stimulation that coffee provides, and her coffee is black—the stronger, the better. For another patient coffee is social. She savors the morning ritual of going to the coffee shop, "where somebody knows your name." For a third patient, coffee is nurturing. She leaves home each morning with the coffee her spouse has brewed for her the same as he has done each day for the past twenty years. How could she possibly turn it down? That'd be like breaking up, no? For a fourth patient, coffee is relaxing. It's the "break" in "coffee break" that she can't give up. Going for coffee gets her out of the office, plain and simple. And for a fifth patient, coffee is a treat that satisfies a sweet craving. She chooses a coffee *drink;* she's probably okay with switching to decaf, in fact, she'd likely be happy with any drink that's sweet and covers the taste of the coffee—a taste she doesn't really even enjoy.

Many different reasons, yet tell any of these folks they can't have "their coffee" and they're all bound to cringe, possibly walk out the door, and never return. Similarly, try to give them each the same replacement, and my rate of compliance only improves marginally. So you see, each coffee drinker needs *her* replacement. In fact, that replacement may need to evolve as weeks go by. (Think large to medium to small, and then eventual decrease to none at all.) Take a moment to think about what influences *your* need.

THE USUAL SUSPECTS	A.K.A.	THE POTENTIAL THREAT(S)	HEALTHY EXCHANGES
Alcohol	Wine, beer, liquors, mixed drinks, and sauces containing alcohol	Irritation and inflammation of the digestive tract with routine consumption and/or overconsumption (Note: Some alcoholic beverages contain gluten.)	Limit frequency and quantity (one serving per occasion— 4 ounces wine, 1 ounce liquor) Avoid beer and carbonated mixers; they're a double whammy.
			Learn to sip and taste as desired/tolerated. Instead of a pre- or post-meal drink, try gentian root (bitters) — nature's digestif—before or after meals.
			Schedule meetings as walks, meals, tea shops and social outings for spas, salons, movies, etc. to remove the temptation and pressure to drink.
Wheat	Wheat berry, wheat flour, seitan, wheat bran, and food products containing these ingredients	Many people with IBS demonstrate wheat sensitivity/intolerance.	Try other types of fiber, grains, and flours. The "other" grains are packed with nutrients (including protein) and make great-tasting substitutions for wheat. If you are going to have wheat, do so less often and go for the best quality. Wheat bran is not advised for IBS sufferers.

THE USUAL SUSPECTS	A.K.A.	THE POTENTIAL THREAT(S)	HEALTHY EXCHANGES
Caffeinated beverages	Regular coffee, caffeinated soda, and black, oolong, and green teas (Note: Decaf coffee appears to irritate the digestive system, albeit to a lesser extent, than regular coffee.)	As a stimulant caffeine stimulates contractions in the digestive tract (as well as of the arteries, which can help trigger symptoms of headaches, cramps, etc.). Both regular and decaf coffee contain acids that are irritating to the digestive tract. Routine consumption can create a dependency on the beverage (for energy, for bowel movement, etc.). Drinking instead of eating a meal, especially breakfast (on an empty stomach), is likely to further irritate the digestive tract.	Start by drinking less at one time or less often. Dilute it with ice cubes or a milk replacement. Taper down—Switch to half-decaf half regular coffee or black to green to white to naturally-decaffeinated tea. Try an herbal tea with healing properties, such as chamomile and peppermint. Try Teecino or other coffee replacements. Get stimulated naturally. Figure out why you need the stimulant. Eat a digestion-friendly snack or meal before or with your beverage to help you consume less and diminish its irritation to the digestive tract.
Carbonation	Mineral waters, sodas, fruit drinks, and beer	Bubbles in equals bubbles out (flatulence).	Try herbal teas, water with small amounts of fruit juice or lemon/lime. Let the carbonated drink become flat.
Chocolate	Cocoa, chocolate-flavored products, and milk chocolate	Caffeine (see above) Milk (see below) Contains magnesium, which relaxes muscles like the digestive tract so it may exacerbate some IBS symptoms (diarrhea) but help others (motility and cramping).	Try small amounts. Choose high cocoa content (70% or greater). Avoid those with milk fat, casein, sugar alcohols (especially sugar-free products), high fructose corn syrup, and partially hydrogenated oils

THE USUAL SUSPECTS	A.K.A.	THE POTENTIAL THREAT(S)	HEALTHY EXCHANGES
Saturated fat and fried foods	Red meat, egg yolk, bacon, sausage, battered foods at restaurants (such as potatoes, vegetables, and calamari), coconut oil, butter, cream, cheese, and mayonnaise	Greater intake of less healthy fats (and any intake of the unhealthy ones) versus healthy and essential ones contributes to a number of chronic diseases and symptom exacerbation. These foods require longer digestion, increasing risk of irritation within the digestive tract.	Use healthy fats (such as olive oil, avocado, nuts, and seeds) routinely to provide nutrient balance at meals. Ensure adequate consumption of essential fatty acids (such as ground flaxseeds, fish and fish oil, and walnuts). Limit quantity and frequency of these foods. Aim for the highest quality—grass-fed, hormone-free animals (and their products), and DHA-fortified yolks.
Fruits, vegetables, and legumes	Brussels sprouts, cabbages, broccoli, cauliflower, kale, radish, turnip, rutabaga, garlic, onions, cucumbers, celery, apples, prunes, beans, including soy and peanuts (Note: While these are gas makers, the recipes and suggestions outline ways to eat these very nutritious foods and reduce their gas-making potential.)	These foods may cause gas and bloating.	Lightly cook fruits and vegetables. Initially consume small quantities with more easily digestible fruits and vegetables. Pre-soak beans. Cook with fennel or caraway seeds. Puree beans, fruit, and vegetables for improved tolerance. Combine with a small amount of healthy fat (such as olive oil and avocado). Introduce gradually in small amounts. Start with the small beans (aduki, mung, lentils), which tend to be more easily digested.
Night shades	Potato, tomato, eggplant, all peppers (except black), chilies, and paprika	Certain people are night shade-sensitive and may see an improvement in their symptoms with a trial elimination.	Trial elimination for those who also suffer from headaches, arthritis, rheumatoid arthritis, chronic diarrhea. Cooking these vegetables and adding miso, seaweed, salt, and parsley may reduce the negative effect.

THE USUAL SUSPECTS	A.K.A.	THE POTENTIAL THREAT(S)	HEALTHY EXCHANGES
Sugar alcohols and Monosodium glutamate	Ingredients ending in –ol, especially malitol and sorbitol. MSG has many names and may be found in some hydrolyzed veg-etable proteins.	Sugar alcohols are meant to be indigestible and as such can cause flatulence and cramping of the digestive tract. MSG can cause gastrointestinal symptoms in MSG-sensitive individuals.	Eat and drink foods, not food products. Avoid sugar-free gum and mints. Use natural sweeteners like stevia (try because for some it can be an irritant), agave nectar, honey, and blackstrap molasses. Avoid foods containing MSG.
Dairy	Milk, butter, cream, and yogurt	Getting enough calcium from non-dairy sources. Calcium is one of several nutrients needed for bone health. Some dietary modifications will improve calcium retention (i.e., caffeine increases calcium *loss*, alcohol *inhibits* calcium absorption, high sodium diets increase calcium *loss*).	Consume non-dairy calcium sources such as teff, buck-wheat, tofu, carob, fortified non-dairy milk substitutes, beans, molasses, dried figs, seeds, cooked greens, and seaweed.
Milk	All products con-taining casein, including sherbet or ice milk	After about 5 years old, many people can no longer success-fully digest lactose. Some peo-ple have sensitivities or allergies to milk proteins (especially casein). Milk protein can increase mucus production.	Drink Lactaid milk or take a lactase enzyme before eating. Choose low-fat or skim Lactaid. Try milk replacements without casein and *preferably* without carageenan, such as rice, soy, oat, and almond milks.
Yogurt and fermented dairy	Yogurts from differ-ent animals, soy-bean, rice options	Milk protein allergy or sensitiv-ity. Added sugars are a favorite food of bad bacteria. Natural yogurt is a good source of good bacteria.	Avoid processed frozen yogurts, which may contain sugar alcohols. Try a natural, plain yogurt or fermented dairy product by itself or with well-tolerated fruits or vegeta-bles to see how your system responds.

THE USUAL SUSPECTS	A.K.A.	THE POTENTIAL THREAT(S)	HEALTHY EXCHANGES
Butter and cream	Includes ice cream, foods sautéed in butter, sour cream, and butter and cream sauces	See "milk" section. Has a high amount of saturated fat.	Butter can be replaced with oils, nut and seed butters, fruit butters, avocado, applesauce, and non-butter spreads—all creating different twists on old favorites or making new favorites. Again, read the labels for potential irritants and remember to avoid hydrogenated oils (trans fats). What to do on a warm summer day instead of enjoying ice cream? Check out the dessert section for dairy-free options as potential new favorites.
Cheese	Cheeses from different animals, such as cow, sheep, and goat. Read labels for casein.	See "milk" section. Has a high fat content. (Note: A high-fat content means that it stays in the gut longer and generates more irritation to the digestive system.)	Cheese replacements do exist and may satisfy on occasion. Goat cheese and sheep's milk cheeses, in small quantities, appear to be better tolerated than their cow's milk equivalents. (Read the label as many people assume a cheese like feta is from goat's milk, which is not necessarily true.) Hard cheeses may be better tolerated. Try options based on what satisfies: If it's the melted, creamy mouth feel you're looking for, a creamy spread of nuts or avocado may do the trick. Conversely, if it's something for the top of a salad or soup, vegetable shavings, croutons, nuts, or seeds may be a better match.

The Extras: The Top TEN (Truly Essential Nutrients)

In cooking school or class, one of the first assignments is the herb and spice lab. Here students learn the value of using herbs and spices to better develop recipes. Because herbs and spices are usually called for in sometimes seemingly miniscule amounts, a cooking novice may wonder if a certain spice is *really* necessary, may choose to skip over it, and may ultimately bear the consequences with a less appealing end product. Have you ever gone to make a recipe and not had the spice, decided to make it anyway, and experienced firsthand a subtle absence or a significant off-taste to your finished product? Perhaps, when dining out, you've tried to make up for a spice-deficient dish by adding a sauce, only to find that after heaping on the sauce it merely disguises the poor-tasting dish below? If you can relate to any of these experiences, you already know the crucial role of herbs and spices. They unleash the tastes, texture, and even appearance of your main ingredients, as well as add their own marks of distinction.

In this book, herbs and spices are the Top TEN, or Truly Essential Nutrients. You may be surprised, or not, to learn that they're not foods at all. Yet, like herbs and spices do for main ingredients in a recipe, the Top TEN unleash the healing properties of food and help to engage all your senses for optimal healing and overall health. In many of our lives, the Top TEN, nutrients L, M, N, O, P, Q, R, S, T, U are deficient to varying degrees, underutilized, and overshadowed despite awareness that they are essential to our health. *Recipes for IBS* calls for bringing these key nutrients back into the mix, as an integral part of the recipe. Here are the Top TEN:

- **NUTRIENT L—LAUGHTER:** Laughter is therapy. I love to quote Jimmy Buffet, "If we couldn't laugh, we'd all go insane." True. Laughing not only relaxes us, it brings in more oxygen to our systems, strengthens our core muscles, and encourages the release of negative energy, all of which ultimately reduce the burden of stress on our bodies. Laugh at your errors, at the driver that cuts you off, at the next machine voice with whom you're forced to "talk" for customer service. Laugh big, laugh hard, laugh again and again. It's free, it's easy, and it's, well, fun. So why not laugh a little. And if you can't find anything funny these days, laugh at how ridiculous that is ...

- **NUTRIENT M—MASSAGE:** Touch heals. Massage has many forms—from a loved one or a practitioner, from totally passive and nurturing to very active and intentionally draining, at your home or at a spa, etc. Discover massage and its healing power.

- **NUTRIENT N—NURTURE YOU:** Learning to nurture yourself is critical to healing. Often, by demand or desire, individuals prioritize nurturing others over themselves, resulting in inappropriate deflection of attention away from the self. This behavior can be intentional or unintentional with the same result. Nurturing yourself requires identifying experiences or things that bring you back to your connection with yourself. Nurturing yourself does not necessarily demand moments of isolation, yet the value of time alone can't be overstated. Take time every few days or each week to plan for activities (or lack thereof) that will help you to nurture yourself.

- **NUTRIENT O—OXYGEN:** Does the fact that we'd be dead without oxygen adequately express the value of this nutrient? Despite being born with the ability, many of us fail to adequately breathe throughout the day. This failure has actual and severe health repercussions over time. Digestion alone requires oxygen to facilitate the reactions involved with garnering energy from food and allocating nutrients. Taking time out to breathe and learn proper breath work should be a vital part of your prescription for healing.

- **NUTRIENT P—PHYSICAL ACTIVITY:** Physical activity is different than exercise. Physical activity is the umbrella which covers the broad spectrum of ways to move the body, ranging from highly relaxing to very rigorous. Daily physical activity is critical for our bodies and spirits. But it is equally critical to match your physical activity with your body's and soul's needs in that moment. For example, if you're running on three hours of sleep, you may benefit more from a yoga class or a massage coupled with an early night to bed, than trying to fit in a run or spinning class, which calls on your body's virtually non-existent reserves in that moment. Conversely, if your client's demands worked you to the brink of exploding, heading to the gym for some running or shadow boxing (think of your client's face) before you go home, or eat, may be the perfect match. I often suggest keeping a nutrient P journal for a month to see if you're challenging yourself to achieve variety as well as frequency.

- **NUTRIENT Q—QUIET:** It may be our most precious and endangered natural resource. Many of us experience ongoing audio assaults—both of our choosing and those beyond our control—routinely throughout our day. I challenge you to develop a plan to minimize audio assaults within your control. Retreat to a quiet space (which may require making a quiet space first) a few times a week to give your body practice knowing the difference between sound and quiet.

- **NUTRIENT R—RELAXATION:** Stress is not the root of all evil. In fact, stress encourages us to achieve great things and to escape disaster, and it plays a key role in enabling survival. However, the inability to reduce or stop stress, to *relax* your body, depletes the body's reserves, increases the risk for chronic disease, and presents challenges to your digestive system. From our days in the cave, the design of the human body is such that in moments of high stress (think "lions, and tigers, and bears … oh my") energy for proper digestion is halted and diverted to energy for survival—that required to sprint, climb, or scramble away from a predator. This survival advantage exists today; however, today this "advantage" often becomes a "disadvantage" as survival stress becomes chronic stress—that endured daily in the form of environmental stress as well as self-imposed stress. When stress is chronic, the body consistently suffers from suboptimal digestion. Thus, relaxation—the ability to stop stress—becomes a critical component in the treatment of IBS and the promotion of optimal health.   What relaxes is different for us all and in any given moment. I've noted with interest that the discussion of relaxation is often a stressful topic for my patients. I witness physical withdrawal at the mention of yoga, meditation, sleep, time for a walk, et cetera out of fear of failure or lack of free time. I am the first to agree that if you hate an activity or if it stresses you out it's not the relaxation tool for you. However, I don't accept the excuse of not having time to relax. For each person, there is something or several things that enables the body to relax. A bath? Getting your nails done? Taking the dog for a walk? Letting someone else take the dog for a walk while you do some stretches? Having sex? Coloring? Knitting? Swinging on the swings? etc. etc. etc. Similar to the apoplectic look I witness at the onset of the "relaxation" chat, I eagerly await the "I think I can" light bulb at the point when a relaxation suggestion switches on the light and my patient says, "Yeah, I could try that." And with that, I usually see them relax a little. What relaxes you?

- **NUTRIENT S—SLEEP:** Our bodies are built to work, to recover, and to work again. They are also built to respond to light and dark. Today, the use of stimulants (lights, stress, caffeine, television, etc.) present challenges to sleep, which is one of our bodies' best self-healing tools. Sleep is our catch-up time, both emotionally and physically. If you are not sleeping properly or sufficiently (recommendations for which differ individually but fall in the range of 7 to 9 hours nightly), you are cheating your healing efforts.

- **NUTRIENT T—TIME:** Yes, we are all busy. Yes, time is precious. But time is yours. I don't allow patients to tell me, "I don't have time …" I require them to say, "I am having trouble finding the time for…" With all that goes on in lives today, it's not only okay but a really good idea to ask for help if you're having trouble making time for you and your needs. It may require some creative prioritization. But it's there. You can find time.

- **NUTRIENT U—UNDERSTANDING:** Be understanding. To yourself and to others. Understand that it may take time for your digestive system to feel better. Understand that you (or your mom, or your doctor, or your boss) are not to blame for how badly your system has felt at times. Understand that being understanding requires taking time to process how you feel and how others may be feeling, to not act, to not react, but just to be and sense for an understanding. Then you can move forward with confidence that your next move makes sense for you.

INGREDIENT 5

The Finales: The Remedies

The fifth "ingredient" in our recipe for IBS treatment is the remedies: dietary supplements. Have you ever tasted or seen a completed recipe and wondered how in the heck did someone get it to taste or look a certain way? Was it magic? No. It isn't magic, rather it's the combination of using quality basics, the right main ingredients, herbs and spices, and then a little something extra.

What's the extra? Maybe it's a cooking technique they've perfected or a rare variety of a fruit or vegetable. Regardless, of what "it" actually is, it's what the extra represents that's the important concept. The extra is the personal touch that cook adds, something that they've learned to use, that works because they feel comfortable with using it. It isn't magic; it's a tool, and in the hands of a skilled user, it completes the recipe just right.

In *Recipes for IBS,* remedies are the extras. They don't work without quality basics, foods that heal, and the Top TEN. But, when in the hands of a skilled user (a qualified healthcare practitioner) the right remedy can be the "it" that optimizes the healing potential of all the other pieces.

Supplements

Just as the cook didn't use magic, there is no magic pill, I repeat, *no magic pill* when it comes to healing the digestive system. Supplementation—the use of nutrients (in addition to food) or herbs for healing purposes—supplements the healing efforts made in all aspects of your life. I do not endorse taking supplements unless you commit to making dietary and lifestyle modifications as your primary healing strategies.

With their *supplemental* role explained, the supplements identified below are those frequently used by experienced healthcare practitioners to combat the range of IBS symptoms and to promote healing the gut. A word of caution: There are real issues with supplementation, including product quality, dosages, interactions with medications, and contraindications. (See story on page 30.) Remember if something is discussed in a book, magazine, or on television, it is being presented in terms of the masses not the individual. What you need—both product and dosage—should be determined between you and your healthcare provider. For this reason, the following section does not include product names, dosages, or provide specific treatment plans. See the "Resources" section on page 180 for additional information.

- **FIBER:** This helps to bulk the stool, scrub the digestive tract, and enable a hospitable environment for good bacteria. Here are some supplemental fiber sources that work well for IBS patients:
  - Ground flaxseeds (Keep them in an airtight, dark container in the refrigerator or freezer.)
  - Chia seeds
  - Rice bran
  - Oat bran
  - Psyllium (In powdered or capsule forms; avoid products that contain sugar alcohols to make them sugar-free.)

A Story About Supplements

I recently saw a patient who, prior to seeing me, visited her internist with high blood pressure despite a history of medication use that kept her blood pressure well controlled. The internist sent her to a cardiologist immediately, who in turn increased her medication and sent her to me for a discussion of, among other things, dietary factors that can contribute to high blood pressure. Prior to our meeting, I asked her to keep a food log and bring in any supplements she was taking.

At our appointment, I reviewed her diet and her supplements, finding no triggers for recent blood pressure changes and developed her plan to achieve her personal health goals. As is customary, I asked about her bowel function—both current and historically—and that is when something clicked. She mentioned seeing a nutritionist/chiropractor a few years ago who gave her something that "worked beautifully" for her constipation at the time. Her supplement bag contained no laxative type products, but I asked about this old product anyway. "Well, now that you mention it, I was so distraught by the return of the constipation that a few weeks ago I called up that practitioner. I'm no longer his patient but he was nice enough to tell me over the phone how I could order that

supplement from him. It came in the mail, let's see, that was a Saturday, and I took a few, then on Sunday I still wasn't regular so I took several more. I think I took six." I asked her what day she went to the internist. "Monday morning." Then she smiled. "Do you think it had anything to do with my blood pressure?"

We got on the Internet, found the fiber supplement, found that a serving is one tablet (She took 3, then 6), and found an ingredient known for the potential to elevate blood pressure. Ah-ha's for all of us.

That practitioner should not have recommended a product to someone other than a current patient. The patient should have presented a list of supplements (including manufacturer) to her doctors. I needed to ask her to bring in *all* supplements—current and recent past.

This story illustrates how even a fiber supplement can have ingredients that interact negatively with your system. Consult a qualified healthcare practitioner before taking supplements. A store representative does not suffice unless licensed and accepting responsibility for you as a patient, which means taking a full history.

- **FIBER COMBINATIONS:** Some are better than others based on the ingredients. (Avoid wheat bran.) Read the ingredient labels. Some contain fruit skins and pectin to improve taste and texture. This is acceptable for most people.

- **MAGNESIUM:** This mineral helps muscles (including those in your digestive system) to relax. Magnesium balances calcium's constricting nature. Magnesium glycinate is reputedly easiest on the digestive system, but magnesium citrate works well for most and tends to be less expensive and more available.

- **GOOD BACTERIA (PROBIOTICS):** When it comes to bacteria and our digestive system, it's one big competition. The competition for "gut space" occurs between good and bad bacteria. Our digestive system needs enough good bacteria to balance the bad bacteria that will naturally find its way there. With IBS patients, probiotic supplementation may prove quite effective in the reduction of symptoms as the proper balance of bacteria. Additionally, for those with diarrhea, it may be beneficial to experiment with beneficial yeast (see "Resources" section on page 100), in addition to beneficial bacteria. Product type and quality, dosage, and storage are critical when it comes to good bacteria for product effectiveness. Note: Many probiotics sold are not dairy-free, and in my opinion these are not the best choice for IBS patients.

- **FISH OIL (EPA AND DHA):** These essential fatty acids promote health by encouraging the body's production of anti-inflammatory hormones. Product quality is critical here as is product storage and shelf life.

- **OTHERS:** The following other nutrients may help promote healing of the digestive system:
  - Deglycyrrhizinated licorice (DGL)
  - L-glutamine
  - Prebiotics (FOS, larch arabinogalactans, phosphatidylcholine, inulin)
  - Turmeric
  - Digestive enzymes
  - Peppermint oil
  - Ginger
  - Rice protein powders
  - Chamomile, lavender, berry leaf teas
  - Triphala
  - Laxatives, enemas, fasts, flushes and colonics—while there may be a temporary role for these products or treatments, they should be used under the supervision of a healthcare practitioner. This includes senna, aloe vera juice, and other herbal products claiming cleansing properties.

The Right Quantity

Overeating can overwhelm the digestive system. This holds as true for high-quality, nutrient-dense foods as it does for other foods. Indeed, consuming too much of a valuable nutrient, like fiber, can have extremely unpleasant consequences. In order to achieve the goals of symptom management and gut healing, we ideally need your gut to be underwhelmed.

Being underwhelmed doesn't mean under-eating in terms of overall nutrients consumed in a day; rather, it means that for optimal digestion eating smaller and less complicated meals can improve digestion. Here are a few strategies to help your gut stay underwhelmed:

- Aim to spread out your nutrient intake over meals and snacks throughout the day.

- Balance your meals with representatives from each of the major nutrient categories (carbohydrates, proteins, and fats) and add non-starchy vegetables as often as possible.

- Several factors—including your life stage, activity level, and body composition—impact nutrient needs, so individual recommendations should be made by a qualified health-care practitioner working with you to achieve your goals.

- I find the range of 1 to 2 servings per eating occasion from each group C-P-F, which stands for carbohydrate-protein-fat, (see the "Food Form" on page 33) with unlimited quantities of non-starchy vegetables per meal appropriate for most individuals.

- Snacks can be a mini-meal, a single serving from one group plus non-starchy vegetables or just non-starchy vegetables.

- Increase fiber intake, but gradually, ideally by adding small amounts of fibrous foods to meals or snacks.

- Measure portions at home a few times so that you can better approximate appropriate portions when eating outside of the home.

- Let your gut wake up relaxed and go to bed relaxed as well. Eating too much, too soon in the morning can upset a sensitive digestive system. Similarly, eating too close to bedtime can prevent the digestive system from finishing its work in time to relax and take needed time off.

Food Form

The following chart helps to identify the main nutrients in the foods we eat daily. Use this chart in conjunction with the discussion on quantity (see section on left) to effectively plan eating occasions with nutrient balance, which will optimally support your digestion and metabolism.

	GRAINS	LEGUMES	STARCHY VEGETABLES	FRUIT	NUTS AND SEEDS	OILS	PROTEINS	NON-STARCHY VEGETABLES
Carbohydrates	✖	✖	✖	✖				Considered
Proteins		✖			✖		✖	free foods.
Fats					✖	✖		Eat often.

	GRAINS (C) (75–100 calories)	LEGUMES (C,P) (100–1200 calories)	STARCHY VEGETABLES (C) (45–60 calories)	FRUIT (C) (75–90 calories)
Portion	1 slice, a piece about the size of your palm, or ½ cup cooked (Look for approximately 15 grams total carbohydrate, less than 5 grams of sugar, and more than 3 grams fiber.)	½ cup cooked, ¼ cup spreads, ¾ cup soups, 1 cup (8 oz.) (for tofu), or the size of a small fist	½ cup cooked, ½ medium (for sweet potato), 2 medium (for carrots), or 12 mini (for baby carrots)	See individual fruits below.
Foods	Oats, rice (except white), quinoa, amaranth, millet, buckwheat, barley, bulgur, spelt, teff, kamut, crackers, bread, tortilla, and pancake	Beans, hummus, peas, tofu, peanuts	Winter squashes, sweet potato, beets, carrots, turnip, parsnip, rutabaga	1 medium apple, pear, or orange; ½ banana; 2 small tangerines, plums, apricots, nectarines or plums; 1 cup berries; 2 figs or dates; 15 grapes or cherries; ½ grapefruit; ¼ medium melon

	ANIMAL PROTEINS (P) (130–160 calories)	NUTS AND SEEDS (F,P) (90–110 calories)	FATS AND OILS (F) (80–100 calories)	NON-STARCHY VEGETABLES (10–25 calories)
Portion	4–5 ounces prepared, a piece about the size of your palm, 3 egg whites, 1 small can in water	8–15 nuts (bigger nut = fewer; smaller nut = more), 1 tablespoon nut and seed butters, 2 tablespoons seeds	1 tablespoon, ¼ avocado, 8–10 olives	Considered free
Foods	Fish, egg whites, chicken breast, turkey, lean pork, leg of lamb, buffalo	Walnuts, pistachios, almonds, pine nuts, flaxseeds, sesame seeds, pumpkin seeds, macadamia nuts, cashews, pecans, hazelnuts, brazil nuts	Olives, avocado, walnut oil, olive oil, canola oil, flaxseed oil, grape seed oil, almond oil Spreads	All vegetables not listed under starchy and prepared as best tolerated.

YOUR FLOUR OPTIONS

TYPE OF FLOUR	USES AND TIPS
Amaranth	This flour has a tangy, spiced flavor, and it's delicious in flatbreads.
Barley	Try this flour in pancakes and cookies, though it's best combined 50/50 with another flour, such as oat. It may make a stickier dough (require more of the dry ingredients such as flour than the original recipe called for).
Buckwheat	Combine this flour 50/50 with rice or oat flour and use it to make breads or pancakes.
Chestnut	This light, creamy flour is great in cakes, cookies, puddings, and soups.
Corn meal	Try corn meal in light breads, muffins, and scones.
Garbanzo	This flour has a strong flavor, but I like it in sauces and spreads. It's best combined 50/50 with another flour for a more desirable flavor.
Kamut	Breads and baked goods are delicious with this flour. It can also replace wheat flour in baked goods.
Millet	This flour is coarse, so it may require more liquid. Always combine it with another flour, using one-third millet to two-thirds other flour.
Oat	Light, this flour is good for creating moistness in baked goods, such as breads, cookies, crusts, and pastries.
Rye	While it may make a stickier dough, this flour is good for breads.
Soy	Because it has a strong flavor, use this flour in small amounts and with spices to cover its flavor.
Sweet rice	This flour adds sweetness and a smoother texture to mochi and puddings.
Teff	Light, gritty, use this flour for flatbreads or desserts in combination with other flours.

Goals and Strategies

The French term, *mise en place,* meaning "everything put in place," is a standard process among chefs. It refers to the organization and preparation that enables an efficient and productive cooking environment. A chef takes the time to review and discuss the recipe, assigns tasks, and allocates tools. This is the point in *Recipes for IBS*—to identify goals, assign strategies, and offer tools. Let's talk about each in turn.

GOAL: Identify your symptoms. As discussed earlier, symptoms of IBS may vary greatly from one individual to the next. Indeed, the same symptom can even result from dramatically distinct causes. For example, with "constipation" as a diagnosis, is it lack of fiber, a question of motility, the result of medication use, the lack of water, etc.? In each case the healing recommendations would be different—perhaps significantly. For example, I never ask a constipation-motility patient to increase fiber initially because adding bulk into a gut that's not moving appropriately is bound to do more damage than good.

STRATEGIES:

- Keep a journal of your symptoms.

- Identify symptom triggers, such as timing, stress, and food.

- Review past and present supplements or medications and their effect on your |digestive tract.

GOAL: Manage your IBS symptoms: Our next goal is to reduce the intensity and frequency of your symptoms.

STRATEGIES:

- Learn to avoid common traps. (See "The Tools" on page 37.)
- Use the tools to begin making appropriate choices for your symptoms.
- Begin making lifestyle modifications. (Review "The Top TEN" on page 26.)
- Plan your plan. Healing takes a commitment. Here are some strategies to help you commit.

Believe in you, yes you can. Embrace healing yourself with a positive attitude despite weeks, months, and even years of disappointment and frustration.

Manage your expectations. It didn't happen overnight, it won't heal overnight. Give yourself, your healthcare practitioner, and any dietary and lifestyle modifications, as well as remedies, the time they need to work. Note that medication works fairly quickly. I believe that our use of medication as a tool has created expectations for immediate results. Such expectations require modification when looking at the entire healing package—dietary, lifestyle, and supplementation remedies. Take it slow and steady. You'll get to your finish line at the right time for you.

Try and try. Acknowledge the power of trial. Recall the "yes you can" attitude discussion. Trying new foods, cooking preparations, and lifestyle modifications will not always feel comfortable. Try and see. But also respect yourself enough to pass on what doesn't appeal (after trying) to you, what is ineffective (after appropriate time), and certainly, on what causes any distress.

Abandon perfection as a concept. Think silver medal or A-/ B+ when it comes to setting your goals, and you're more likely to achieve and sustain them. In my opinion perfection has no place in the discussion of health. I've seen a few too many clients dealing with digestive disturbance linked to seeking "perfect" health regimes and the stress associated with trying to maintain such plans. Conversely, I've seen clients fail out the door, overwhelmed by the prospect of implementing grandiose changes. From beef twice daily to vegan tomorrow, from 2 grams of fiber to 20 per meal—no way. Extreme changes are less sustainable and typically bear negative consequence, such as frustration, worsening of symptoms, or creating new symptoms. That's not what you need. Learn to crawl, then walk, then skip, then jog, then run, then race. You get the idea.

As symptoms diminish (or change), expand your choices to increase the health value of your IBS nutrition plan. For example, as your system starts to feel better you should try moving from cooked to fresh fruit, or incorporating gas makers such as cooked vegetables or beans (according to the recommendations on page 33) to diminish unpleasant side effects.

GOAL: Heal the gut: Learning to manage your IBS symptoms may feel like winning the battle. In reality, it's the achievement of the first two of three goals. The ultimate goal is to heal your digestive system. The strategies in the first two goals help to reduce symptoms (delightful), but equally important, they help prevent new irritation to the system and allow the body to focus its energies on healing itself.

STRATEGIES:

- Manage your IBS symptoms *first*. The body cannot focus on healing itself when allocating the bulk of its resources to fight new irritation.
- Don't get *a* prescription; get *your* prescription. Be it for acupuncture, therapy, supplements, herbs, or medications, your efforts should involve individual attention from a qualified healthcare practitioner(s) who *prescribes* your *personalized* plan.

The Tools

Having the right tools available improves efficiency and effectiveness in cooking. The tools required for *Recipes for IBS* include the color code, the recipes, the sample menus, and the resources.

THE COLOR CODE

Each recipe in this book includes codes that show which symptoms the recipe is helpful to prevent or treat. Using the color code, choose foods appropriate for the prevention and reduction of your symptoms. In some recipes, modifications are listed alongside the color code to help make the recipe more conducive to treating that symptom. Here are the codes:

RED ●: These recipes help with loose stools and diarrhea, with symptoms including urgency associated with uncontrollable evacuation, unformed stools, food allergies or intolerances, and low fiber intake.

GREEN ◉: These recipes help with constipation dealing with fiber, with symptoms including stringy stools, foul-smelling stools or gas during evacuation, and low dietary fiber intake (high protein diets, processed grains, insufficient fruits and vegetables).

BLUE ◉: These recipes help with constipation dealing with motility and lubrication, with symptoms including the inability to evacuate at all or fully despite feeling the need, stool coming out as small pellets, lower abdominal pressure, and sufficient (or even high) fiber intake not resolving problem. Additional complaints include migraines or skin irritations, and taking multiple medications.

ORANGE ◎: These recipes help with indigestion, with symptoms including flatulence/gas (especially foul-smelling), bloating, cramps, pressure, rumbling, sufficient (or even high) fiber intake not resolving problem, and complaints of food allergies or intolerances commonly associated with recent or historic antibiotic use.

PURPLE ◉: These recipes help with really bad days, which may present with diarrhea or constipation. Aptly named, these are the days when symptoms are at their worst.

A WORD FROM THE CHEF

Working with IBS patients, the most frequent questions I receive are, "Can you tell me how to make that?" and "My kids only eat ___, my husband needs to eat _____, and now you're telling me to eat _____. I don't have time to make three meals every time we sit down, is there anything I can serve that works for all of us?" Common excuses I hear are "I've never cooked for myself before," "I have only a really small kitchen," and certainly, "I don't have time to *make* something."

Any of these sound familiar? The recipe selection featured in this book seeks to address these questions and comments so that each reader can find a few go-to or staple options on which to rely, as well as additional choices to investigate when time, effort, and interest allow. These recipes adapt basics and favorites to become not just *appropriate* but *ideal* for the reduction and prevention of IBS symptoms. They *all* were made, at least once, in a small kitchen, using basic kitchen appliances and tools. They were made by me; by my patients, family, and friends; by cooking novices; and by a few true culinary experts—all people whose jobs, hobbies, and familial obligations place constraints on cooking time.

Several willing and critical mouths tasted the recipes giving valuable *feed*back; their comments provide you with an opinion other than my own. Having other people sample, test, re-test, and re-sample the recipes proved invaluable to me in assembling a collection whose goal is to offer something for everyone. Many recipes required numerous trials, and several were ultimately discarded because, despite offering health benefits, they never became palate-pleasing.

"I have indigestion, and after sampling all, and I mean all *(the recipes at the tasting), I feel great!"*

—Donald

CHAPTER 2

The Principles:
Vegetarian and Nonvegetarian Entrees

These are your main dishes. Some days they are a meal in of themselves, at other times they combine perfectly with a supporting cast, extra, or a finale. There's no rule about when you eat a certain recipe during the day. For example, try eggs for dinner and fish for breakfast. Test it out and see how your system responds.

Calming Congee ●◎

◎ *(diarrhea)*

A Chinese breakfast favorite, congee digests easily, making it most useful for those really bad days. With the addition of carrots and ginger powder, this congee helps combat diarrhea, flatulence, and general indigestion. Caution: Don't judge a book by its cover; once you experience the healing powers of this "ugly" dish, you're bound to see its inner beauty.

INGREDIENTS

- 1 cup (190 g) uncooked brown rice
- 4 large carrots, sliced
- 2 tablespoons (11 g) powdered ginger
- 5 cups (1175 ml) water

In a deep sauce pot, place the rice, carrots, ginger, and water. Cover and simmer on low heat for at least 4 hours. Remove from the heat and serve warm.

YIELD: Makes 4 servings.

NUTRITIONAL ANALYSIS
Per Serving: 212 Calories; 2g Fat (trace saturated fat); 5g Protein; 45g Carbohydrate; 3g Dietary Fiber; 0mg Cholesterol; 37mg Sodium.

Millet Marvel Congee ●◎◎

◎ *(diarrhea)*

With a reputation for calming morning sickness and being anti-fungal, millet distinguishes itself as a highly alkalinizing, gluten free grain.

INGREDIENTS

- ¼ cup (50 g) uncooked millet
- 1¼ cups (295 ml) water
- 1 cup (115 g) cubed winter squash, such as acorn
- ½ daikon radish or other radish, chopped
- 2 teaspoons mustard powder
- ½ cup chopped fennel

In a deep saucepot, place the millet, water, squash, radish, mustard powder, and fennel. Cover and simmer on low for at least 4 hours, stirring occasionally. Remove from heat and serve warm.

YIELD: Makes 4 servings.

NUTRITIONAL ANALYSIS
Per Serving: 72 Calories; 1g Fat (trace saturated fat); 2g Protein; 14g Carbohydrate; 3g Dietary Fiber; 0mg Cholesterol; 19mg Sodium.

NOTES

You can buy daikon radishes at Oriental markets.

Fennel is also called anise.

QuintesSensual Quinoa

○ *sprinkle flaxseeds or chia seeds to add fiber* ● *omit walnuts and replace blueberries with blackberries and/or a less-ripe banana*

A true meal satisfies nutrient needs as well as the senses. This dish offers a combination of textures, scents, and colors to provide ample stimulation for your senses. Easily digestible quinoa is an excellent staple for IBS patients because it is gluten-free and a good source of quality protein, calcium, and other vitamins and minerals. Here, ginger and mint offer additional digestive support.

INGREDIENTS

- ⅓ cup raw quinoa (per package directions you may want to rinse and dry it before using)
- ½ cup (25 g) fresh mint leaves, minced
- 1 teaspoon ground ginger
- ¼ teaspoon salt
- 1 cup water
- 2 tablespoons (28 ml) toasted walnut oil
- 3 tablespoons (45 ml) fresh lime juice
- 1 cup (145 g) blueberries or coarsely chopped cherries
- ½ cup (65 g) chopped walnuts

In a dry frying pan, lightly toast the quinoa for 1 to 2 minutes. Remove from the heat and combine with the mint, ginger, and salt.

In a large 2-quart (2-L) saucepan, bring the water and quinoa mixture to a boil. Reduce the heat to a simmer, cover, and cook for 6 to 8 minutes, until the water is fully absorbed and the quinoa is light and fluffy.

Meanwhile, in a cup, whisk together the oil and lime juice.

Pour the quinoa from the saucepan into a mixing bowl; fold the blueberries or cherries and nuts into the quinoa. Pour the dressing over the quinoa mixture and combine well. You may serve this warm or cold by allowing it to chill for at least 1 hour (better if overnight).

YIELD: Makes 4 servings.

NUTRITIONAL ANALYSIS

Per Serving: 238 Calories; 17g Fat (1 g saturated fat); 6g Protein; 19g Carbohydrate; 3g Dietary Fiber; 0mg Cholesterol; 144mg Sodium.

NOTE

Fennel is also called anise.

"It's great—some crunch, yet smooth and light. I'd like it for breakfast or after a workout."

—Pete

● Loose Stools & Diarrhea ○ Fiber ◉ Motility and Lubrication ◎ Indigestion ◉ Really Bad Days

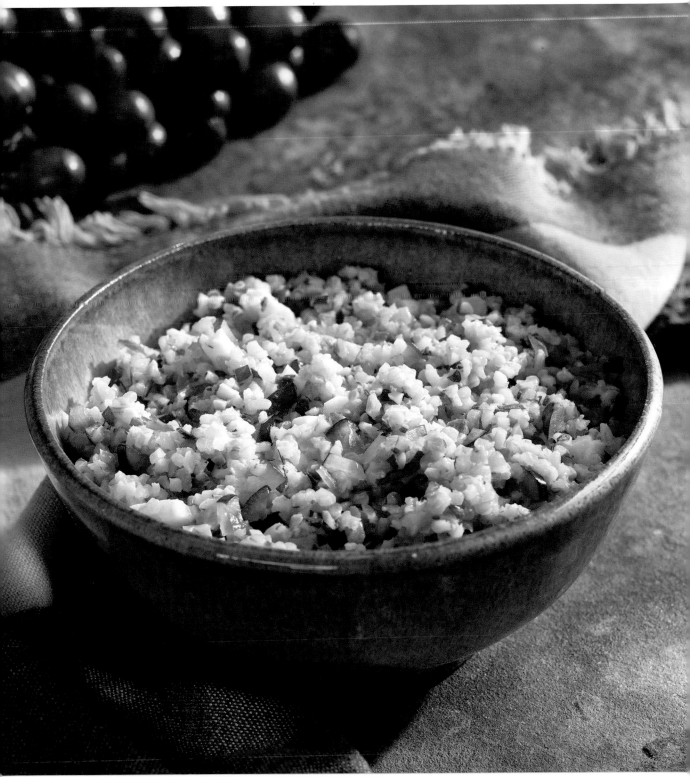

Hot Vegetable Pie °◎

Warm and filling, this recipe makes an excellent breakfast or dinner on a cold day. For digestive success, it combines two techniques: cooking the vegetables and adding caraway seeds, which reduce the gas-making potential of some healthful foods such as cauliflower, onion, and garlic.

INGREDIENTS

- 1 pie crust (8- or 9-inch, or 20- or 22.5-cm) of your choice (try the Quinoa Crust on page 156)
- ½ cauliflower head (or 2 cups frozen, or 265 g)
- 3 cups (90 g) greens, stems removed (such as collards, spinach, or chard)
- ¼ pound (115 g) fresh mushrooms
- 1 tablespoon (14 ml) canola oil or grapeseed oil, divided
- 1 sweet onion, diced
- 1 clove garlic, minced
- 2 cups (475 ml) milk replacement (try the Curried Nut Milk recipe on page 140, or use store bought rice, almond, or oat 'milk')
- ⅓ cup (50 g) oats
- ¾ cup (85 g) crumbled goat cheese or sheep's milk cheese (strong flavor)
- 3 teaspoons caraway seeds

Preheat the oven to 425°F (220°C, gas mark 7).

Prepare the pie crust and press it into a pie pan.

Steam the cauliflower and greens until soft. (If using a double pot steamer, place the cauliflower closer to the boiling water, otherwise you may want to steam the cauliflower for a few minutes then add the greens.)

In a frying pan, sauté the mushrooms in ½ tablespoon (7 ml) of the oil over medium heat, until they soften. Pile the cauliflower, greens, and mushrooms into the pie crust and set aside.

Oil the frying pan again with the remaining ½ tablespoon (7 ml) of the oil and sauté the onions and garlic, until they begin to soften.

Meanwhile, in a cup, blend the milk replacement with oats, then combine the mixture in the frying pan with the onions and garlic. Cook for 1 to 2 minutes, stirring constantly, to thicken. Remove from the heat and stir in the cheese. Pour over the vegetables in the pie crust. Bake, uncovered, for 25 to 30 minutes. Sprinkle the caraway seeds on top and serve.

"This is cozy like a blanket; a warm, chewy, delicious blanket that is."

—Alison

YIELD: Makes 8 (1-slice) servings.

NUTRITIONAL ANALYSIS

Per Serving: 396 Calories; 20g Fat (4 g saturated fat); 15g Protein; 44g Carbohydrate; 8g Dietary Fiber; 11 mg Cholesterol; 62mg Sodium.

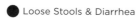 Loose Stools & Diarrhea   Fiber   Motility and Lubrication   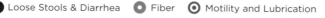 Indigestion   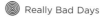 Really Bad Days

Gnocchi Sweet Gnocchi plain or with sprouted sunflower seeds

with flaxseeds or chia seeds and nuts *with sesame oil or black sesame seeds and pine nuts* *(diarrhea) plain*

A truly sweet twist on potato gnocchi, these are wheat-free, naturally sweet, moist, and easily digested. Served with ground flax or hemp seeds or some chopped nuts, it's a nice breakfast or brunch alternative that's bound to hit the sweet spot. Cinnamon, a key ingredient, adds delightful scent and flavor, as it goes to work for us with anti-inflammatory properties, limiting the growth of bacteria and yeasts, and improving blood sugar.

INGREDIENTS

- 3 parsnips
- 1 3/4 cups (195 g) buckwheat flour, divided
- 3/4 cup (85 g) oat flour
- 1 teaspoon allspice
- 3 teaspoons cinnamon
- 1 can (15 ounces, or 430 g) pumpkin puree (without additives)
- 1/2 teaspoon salt

"They look a little like logs of wood, so I wasn't expecting much. I was so surprised; they're deliciously sweet and filling. I might want them with a sauce—applesauce or berries."

—Kerry

NOTE

Serve the gnocchi warm with berries and hemp seeds or other chopped nuts. Or, let them cool and place them on a cookie sheet in the freezer; once solid, place in a freezer container and store frozen for up to a month.

Preheat the oven to 400° F (200°C, or gas mark 6).

Using a fork, pierce five to six sets of holes into each parsnip. Place the parsnips directly on the oven rack and bake for about an hour, until the flesh is very soft. Rotate the parsnips once or twice to avoid burning the skin.

In a mixing bowl, combine the 1 cup (110 g) of the buckwheat flour and the oat flour, all spice, cinnamon, and pumpkin.

Fill a saucepan halfway with water; add the salt and place the saucepan on top of the stove to be used later.

When the parsnips are cooked, remove the skin and scrape the flesh away from the cores; dispose of the cores and skins. Place the flesh into a food processor and puree or mash it by hand. Blend the parsnips into the pumpkin mixture. At this point, add some of the reserved buckwheat flour to make the dough less sticky.

Sprinkle some of the reserved buckwheat flour onto a flat surface. Bring the water in the saucepan to a boil. Roll out the dough into 3/4 inch (2 cm) "logs." Pinch off small pieces and press one side flat with the back of a fork. Place 10 to 15 of the gnocchi in the boiling water and let them simmer about 2 minutes, until they float to the top. Remove the gnocchi from the water with a strainer spoon.

YIELD: Makes 12 servings

NUTRITIONAL ANALYSIS
Per Serving: 153 Calories; 2g Fat (trace saturated fat); 5g Protein; 32g Carbohydrate; 7g Dietary Fiber; 0mg Cholesterol; 99mg Sodium.

Mediterranean Tofu Scramble

Chard and sesame are the noteworthy ingredients in this scramble. The gorgeous, deep colors of chard leaves—red and green—are directly proportional to their high phytonutrient content. Sesame seeds and oil are known for natural, mild laxative properties; thus, this is a recommended choice for people battling constipation but not for those with chronic diarrhea.

INGREDIENTS

- ½ cup (120 ml) low-sodium vegetable broth
- 1 (12 ounces, or 340 g) package soft tofu or 12–18 egg whites
- 1 bag (16 ounces, or 455 g) mixed red and green chard, stems removed (small leaves preferable)
- 1 teaspoon dark, unrefined sesame seed oil
- 2 tablespoons (18 g) black sesame seeds, ground
- 3 ounces goat cheese or sheep's milk crumbles (optional)

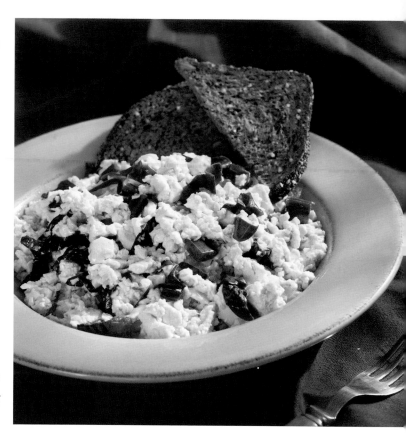

In a sauté pan over medium heat, bring the vegetable broth to a simmer. Add the chard and sauté about 3 to 5 minutes, until wilted. Add the tofu (crumbling with a fork) or egg whites and continue to sauté, stirring frequently. Reduce the heat to medium, add the oil, and sprinkle the seeds, while continuing to stir. Add the cheese, if using, and cover for about 3 minutes. Remove from the heat and place onto plates.

YIELD: Makes 6 servings.

NUTRITIONAL ANALYSIS
Per Serving: 147 Calories; 10g Fat (4 g saturated fat); 11g Protein; 5g Carbohydrate; 2g Dietary Fiber; 15mg Cholesterol; 193mg Sodium.

"Yummmmmm. I am a vegetarian so I did it without the cheese but added some pine nuts. I love the chard; it made it so pretty. I'm taking this with me to a brunch."

—Stacey

SAAG-sational ◉◎●

This Indian dish soothes and satisfies. The spice combination offers anti-bacterial, anti-inflammatory, and anti-flatulence properties. Mustard seeds in particular may help with indigestion and bloating. The slow cooking method helps make these vegetables easily digested as well as delicious.

INGREDIENTS

- 8 ounces (225 g) frozen cauliflower, thawed
- 8 ounces (225 g) frozen, chopped spinach, thawed
- 2 teaspoons ginger powder
- 1 teaspoon fennel seeds
- 1 teaspoon brown mustard seeds
- 1/2 teaspoon chili powder
- 3 teaspoons minced garlic
- 1 teaspoon salt
- 1 red onion, finely chopped
- 1/2 cup (120 ml) grapeseed oil
- 3 teaspoons cilantro
- 15–20 grape tomatoes, halved
- 2–3 tablespoons (28–45 ml) water

Pat the cauliflower dry to remove excess water. Place the spinach in a colander and push the excess water out with back of a mixing spoon.

Using a mortar and pestle (or the back of a spoon), grind the ginger, fennel seeds, mustard seeds, chili powder, garlic, and salt into a thick paste.

In a sauté pan, sauté the onion in the oil, until it softens considerably. Add the spice paste and continue to sauté for a few minutes. Reduce the heat and add the spinach, cilantro, tomatoes, and cauliflower plus the water and continue to cook, stirring frequently. (The dish takes about 20 minutes to cook at this point. The cauliflower should crumble, and the finished dish clumps together with little moisture remaining.)

YIELD: Makes 4 servings.

NUTRITIONAL ANALYSIS
Per Serving: 316 Calories; 28g Fat (3 g saturated fat); 5g Protein; 15g Carbohydrate; 5g Dietary Fiber; 0mg Cholesterol; 603mg Sodium.

"This was way more filling and flavorful than I expected."

—Ted

NOTE

Have a bowl as a meal or partner it with a piece of chicken, fish, or turkey breast.

Crispy Rice Pizza

Oregano, a member of the mint family, provides this recipe with a true pizza flavor, while also helping to reduce flatulence. The addition of goat's milk cheese to the crust imparts flavor tasty enough to give those other stuffed crust pizzas a run for their money.

INGREDIENTS

- ¼ cup (40 g) flaxseeds
- ⅓ cup (75 ml) water
- 3 cups (585 g) cooked brown rice
- 1 red onion, diced
- 1 teaspoon oregano
- 1 teaspoon crushed garlic
- 2 cups (300 g) crumbled goat's milk feta cheese or Parmesan cheese, divided
- 4 mild Italian chicken sausages, or zucchini
- 1 jar (15 ounces, or 430 g) pizza sauce (see note)

Preheat the oven 450° F (230°C, gas mark 8). Coat 13- by 9-inch (32.5- by 22.5-cm) baking pan with canola oil spray.

In a large mixing bowl, soak the flaxseeds in the water for a few minutes. Then whisk them together to form a gel. Mix in the rice, onion, oregano, garlic, and 1 cup of the cheese. Place the mixture in the prepared baking pan. Pat it down to form a crust. Bake for approximately 20 minutes, until lightly browned.

Meanwhile, in a skillet, cook the sausages or zucchini over low heat, rotating each sausage every few minutes. When almost cooked, remove the sausages or zucchinis from the heat and thinly slice.

Remove the crust from the oven. Leave the oven turned on. Spread the sauce onto the crust up to ¼ inch (6 mm) from the edge. Sprinkle the remaining 1 cup cheese evenly on top of the sauce. Arrange the sausage or zucchini over the sauce and cheese. Bake for another 10 minutes. Let cool and cut into 3-inch (7.5 cm) squares to serve.

YIELD: Makes 12 servings.

NUTRITIONAL ANALYSIS

Sausage Pizza: Per Serving: 297 Calories; 20g Fat (8 g saturated fat); 11g Protein; 19g Carbohydrate; 2g Dietary Fiber; 51 mg Cholesterol; 780mg Sodium.
Zucchini Pizza: Per Serving: 175 Calories; 8g Fat (4 g saturated fat); 7g Protein; 20g Carbohydrate; 3g Dietary Fiber; 22mg Cholesterol; 506mg Sodium.

NOTES

If your sauce has garlic and onions in it, eliminate those from the recipe.

This pizza is delicious served on top of steamed, strained pre-cut winter greens.

"This is really, really good. I like the crunchy crust."

—Jim

● Loose Stools & Diarrhea   ◐ Fiber   ◉ Motility and Lubrication   ◎ Indigestion   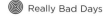 Really Bad Days

Polenta-Broccoli-Pesto Pizza °

Kids find this colorful pizza alternative a tasty treat and fun to make. However, if you keep them out of the kitchen, they may never know they're eating broccoli. You'll love how easy this wheat-free pizza is on your system. Pine nuts, which complete this dish, are one of the richest sources of protein of all nuts, and they're also a mild laxative.

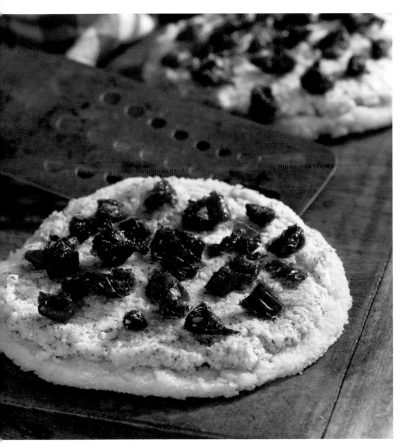

INGREDIENTS

- 2 cups (280 g) uncooked polenta (do not use ready-made)
- 3 cups (275 g) broccoli, steamed
- 1 cup (135 g) pine nuts
- 3 tablespoons (45 ml) olive oil
- 2 cups (220 g) sun-dried tomatoes in oil, diced
- Spray canola or grapeseed oil

Preheat the oven to 350° F (180°C, gas mark 4). Lightly coat a baking sheet or 13- by 9-inch (32.5- by 22.5-cm) pan with cooking spray.

Follow the package directions to prepare the polenta. Spread the polenta thinly onto the prepared pan.

In a food processor, blend the broccoli, pine nuts, and oil, until finely ground. Spread the mixture evenly on top of the polenta. Spread the tomatoes thinly across the broccoli-pesto layer. Bake for 15 to 20 minutes, until lightly browned. Let cool, then cut into squares.

YIELD: Makes 15 servings.

NUTRITIONAL ANALYSIS
Per Serving: 248 Calories; 10g Fat (1 g saturated fat); 7g Protein; 34g Carbohydrate; 5g Dietary Fiber; 0mg Cholesterol; 43mg Sodium.

"My son calls this the 'stoplight' pizza (red, yellow, and green) yet there was no stopping him. When it comes to the taste, this pizza was a 'go.'"

—Sandy
(a.k.a. Mother of Picky Eater)

Heart 'n Colon Porridge

● add fruit and nuts after 40 minutes and continue to simmer for at least another 40 minutes, stirring occasionally

◐ don't toast the barley first ◎● (constipation) without nuts

Oats pack a nutritional power punch, helping to reduce cholesterol, indigestion (especially bloating), and cleanse the colon. Barley, too, helps promote colon and heart health with mild laxative and cholesterol-lowering properties. Some recipes call for toasting barley first, which releases its wonderful aroma. But that is not recommended for individuals suffering from constipation.

INGREDIENTS

- 2 cups (475 ml) water
- 1/2 teaspoon salt
- 1/2 cup (90 g) whole barley (sproutable vs. pearl if available)
- 1/2 cup (85 g) oat groats
- 1/4 cup (60 ml) maple syrup or agave nectar
- 3 cups (435 g) blueberries
- 1 cup (105 g) chopped almonds

In a deep sauce pot, bring the water, salt, barley, and groats to a boil. Cover and simmer for about 40 minutes, until the grains become tender and the water is partially absorbed. (The mixture should be *slightly* runny at this point.) Stir in the syrup or nectar and continue cooking for 5 minutes. Fold in the blueberries and almonds and cook for another 3 minutes.

YIELD: Makes 6 servings.

NUTRITIONAL ANALYSIS
Per Serving: 321 Calories; 14g Fat (2 g saturated fat); 10g Protein; 43g Carbohydrate; 7g Dietary Fiber; 0mg Cholesterol; 190mg Sodium.

"After this delicious start, I'm ready for a day on the slopes. Then again, I feel so cozy and warm, I might just stay in and read and have a little more."

—Pattie

● Loose Stools & Diarrhea   ◐ Fiber   ◉ Motility and Lubrication   ◎ Indigestion   ◉◉ Really Bad Days

Everything-but-the-Kitchen-Sink Hash

using carrots, yam, leeks, sunflower seeds, and chestnuts

Has this ever happened to you? You know you to take need a trip to the grocery store, but you also know you'll feel better giving yourself (and your family) a warm breakfast to start the day right. Here's the answer: Rifle through the cupboards and refrigerator, pulling out cans, bags, and produce for a delicious and satisfying dish. Ingredients such as water chestnuts and artichoke hearts add texture and taste, as well as being beneficial for the gastrointestinal tract. This recipe calls for toasting the barley before cooking, which is not recommended for constipation sufferers.

INGREDIENTS

- 1½ cups (270 g) barley grits
- 4 cups (940 ml) water
- 1 teaspoon salt
- 2 red onions, chopped
- 8 shallots, diced
- 1 cup (240 g) canned fire-roasted tomatoes
- ½ cup (90 g) cooked spinach
- 1 can (10 ounces, or 280 g) chestnuts, drained
- 1 can (8 ounces, or 225 g) water chestnuts, drained
- 1 can (13 ounces, or 370 g) artichoke hearts, drained
- 1 teaspoon thyme
- 1 teaspoon ginger powder
- 2 tablespoons (28 ml) extra virgin olive oil

In a dry saucepan, place the barley over medium heat. Allow it to cook for 3 minutes, stirring to avoid burning. Turn off the heat.

Meanwhile, in a kettle, bring the water to a boil. Stir the barley as you add in the boiling water; it will froth. Add the salt. Begin cooking over a high heat to bring the barley back to a boil. Once boiling, cover, reduce the heat, and simmer for 10 minutes. Remove the barley from the heat and let stand for another 10 minutes.

Meanwhile, in a sauté pan, sauté the onions and the shallots. Once they soften, add the tomatoes and spinach and continue to cook, stirring frequently. Then add the chestnuts, water chestnuts, artichokes, thyme, and ginger. Cook for about 15 minutes, until well-combined and soft, stirring occasionally to prevent sticking to the bottom of the pan. Remove the vegetable mixture from the heat and blend it into the barley, adding the oil.

Meanwhile, coat the sauté pan with cooking spray. Spread the hash back into the sauté pan, cover, and cook over medium-low heat for about 8 to 10 minutes. (Avoid burning the bottom of the hash by keeping the temperature low.) Turn off the heat and let cool for a minute. Slide a spatula around the edges of the hash and slightly underneath to loosen. Place a baking sheet or other large, flat serving plate on top of the saucepan. Gently flip the pan over, immediately placing the flat surface on the counter top. Cut the hash into wedges and serve.

YIELD: Makes 16 servings.

NUTRITIONAL ANALYSIS

Per Serving: 139 Calories; 2g Fat (trace saturated fat); 3g Protein; 28g Carbohydrate; 4g Dietary Fiber; 0mg Cholesterol; 165mg Sodium.

Rustic French Toast °

In The All New All Purpose Joy of Cooking, an excellent kitchen resource, the authors note, "Americans eat French toast for breakfast, but the French serve it for dessert." By playing around with the ingredients to make it more digestively pleasing, this recipe also reduces the sugar and fat load of a traditional French toast. Rustic French Toast offers a more suitable option for breakfast or brunch.

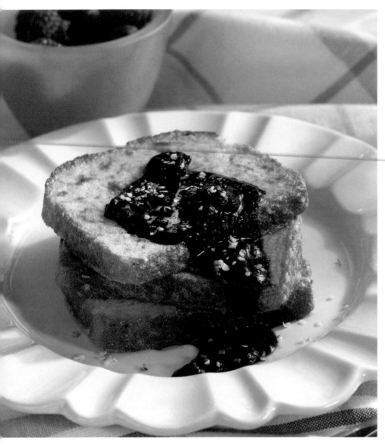

INGREDIENTS

- 1 cup (235 ml) liquid egg whites
- 1 teaspoon cinnamon
- 3/4 cup (175 ml) light, unsweetened coconut milk
- 3/4 cup (175 ml) plain almond milk
- 1 loaf (1 pound, or 455 g) wheat-free bread, sliced thick (see note)
- Hemp-Berry Sauce (page 134)

In a mixing bowl, whisk together the egg whites, cinnamon, coconut milk, and almond milk.

In a shallow storage container with a lid, place the bread and cover with the egg white mixture. Allow the bread to soak in the refrigerator for at least 4 hours (ideally overnight), flipping over once or twice.

Preheat the broiler. Drain the extra liquid from the bread and place the bread on a broiler pan. Broil each side for about 5 minutes, until golden brown. Serve with Hemp-Berry sauce on the side or drizzled over each piece.

YIELD: Makes 6 (1–2 slice) servings.

NUTRITIONAL ANALYSIS
Per Serving: 430 Calories; 19g Fat (7 g saturated fat); 17g Protein; 51 g Carbohydrate; 8g Dietary Fiber; 0mg Cholesterol; 573mg Sodium.

"My favorite! I must have the recipe!"

—Barb

NOTE

I used Julian's rye-quinoa bread, which made about 12 slices.

● Loose Stools & Diarrhea ◉ Fiber ◉ Motility and Lubrication ◎ Indigestion ◎ Really Bad Days

Fruit-tata ◉◉

This meal in a slice appears to be just as well-liked as a dessert. Make it on a Sunday for a crowd, and Monday morning or evening leftovers (if there are any) are sure to please.

INGREDIENTS

- 2 bags (16 ounces, or 455 g, each) frozen berries, including cherries, thawed
- 1 package (16 ounces, or 455 g) egg whites
- 2 tablespoons (28 ml) maple syrup
- 3 teaspoons cinnamon
- 2 cups (310 g) oats
- 2 Fuji apples, peeled
- 2 cups (285 g) raw almonds, finely chopped
- 2 teaspoons vanilla extract

Drain the fruit very well.

In a mixing bowl, whisk the egg whites, maple syrup, vanilla, and cinnamon until well combined. Fold in the oats and refrigerate.

Meanwhile, slice the apples about ¼ inch (6 mm). (Several slices should have a star shape in the middle.) Gently remove the seeds.

Coat a sauté pan with cooking spray. sauté the apples over low heat, flipping them a few times, until golden brown and soft. Remove from the heat.

Take the egg mixture from the refrigerator and gently fold the fruit into the mixture; combine well. Coat a large sauté pan with a cover with cooking spray. Arrange the apple slices to cover the bottom of the pan. Pour the egg-fruit-oat mixture over the apples, cover and cook on low for 5 to 8 minutes. Remove the cover. (The eggs should be formed at this point, not runny.) Spread the almonds evenly on top. Cover and continue to cook for about 3 minutes, until the almonds are held in by the egg mixture. Remove from heat and let cool for a minute. Place a flat serving platter or baking sheet on top of the saucepan. Flip the saucepan so that the fruit-tata lands apples up on the flat surface. Let cool for at least 10 minutes. Cut into wedges and serve.

YIELD: Makes 8 servings.

NUTRITIONAL ANALYSIS
Per Serving: 714 Calories; 22g Fat (2 g saturated fat); 62g Protein; 71 g Carbohydrate; 12g Dietary Fiber; 0mg Cholesterol; 709mg Sodium.

NOTE

You may choose to present this dish before cutting it because it's particularly attractive with the apples on top. Also, you may want to peel off a bit of the egg if it is covering the apples or overly brown.

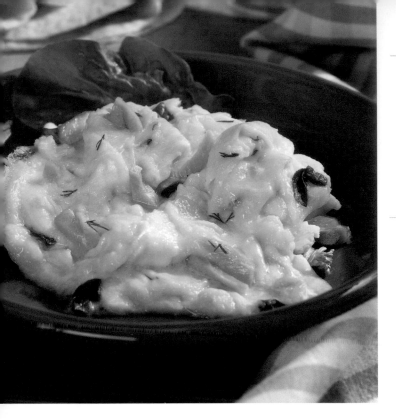

NOTE

This can be eaten alone or served on top of a tortilla.

3 S Scramble ⊙●◎ *add 1 teaspoon dry ginger powder*

Using vegetable broth instead of oil to sauté and scramble imparts this dish with great flavor, and saves calories. Adding fresh dill weed enhances flavor and, equally important, helps settle the digestive system.

INGREDIENTS

- ¹/₂ cup (120 ml) low-sodium vegetable broth
- 1 shallot, peeled and minced (optional)
- 1 package (16 ounces, or 455 g) frozen spinach, thawed and strained
- 16 ounces (475 ml) liquid egg whites or 10 egg whites
- ¹/₄ cup (2 g) fresh dill weed, minced
- 4 ounces (115 g) wild Alaskan smoked salmon, chopped

In a large saucepan, heat the vegetable broth over medium heat. Add the shallot and begin to sauté. After 1 minute, add the spinach, egg whites, and dill, stirring occasionally. As the egg whites become solid, mix in the salmon and cook, covered, for 3 to 5 minutes, until the salmon's color dulls.

YIELD: Makes 4 servings.

NUTRITIONAL ANALYSIS
Per Serving: 133 Calories; 2g Fat (trace saturated fat); 22g Protein; 8g Carbohydrate; 4g Dietary Fiber; 7mg Cholesterol; 564mg Sodium.

Nixed-the-Noodles-for-Spaghetti Pad Thai ◦◎◉

There are no noodles in this dish. For a twist, this pad Thai uses deliciously light spaghetti squash. Add the turmeric for flavor and color, as well as properties that help the body keep its inflammatory response in check.

INGREDIENTS

- 1 spaghetti squash
- 1/4 cup (60 ml) pad Thai sauce (I used Thai Kitchen)
- 3/4 cup (110 g) almonds, chopped
- 1/4 cup (6 g) mint leaves, julienned
- 1/2 cup (120 ml) liquid egg whites or 4 egg whites
- 2 teaspoons turmeric

"I love it. It's great hot. Then I had it the next day cold, and it was just as good."

—Merilee

NOTE

This can be served warm or allowed to cool and then refrigerated overnight and served as a cold salad. You could serve it in the scooped-out spaghetti squash halves.

Preheat the oven to 350 º F (180°C, gas mark 4). Lightly coat a baking sheet with cooking spray.

Cut spaghetti squash in half. (Microwave the squash for a few minutes to soften it if it's difficult to cut uncooked.) Scoop out the seeds.

Place the squash halves cut sides down on the prepared baking sheet. Cover and bake for 45 to 60 minutes. (The squash is done when it's soft enough to take a fork through the flesh and have strings form easily. These will become your "noodles.") Let the squash cool, then use a fork to scrape the flesh of the squash into "noodles." Place the squash noodles in a bowl and toss in the sauce, almonds, and mint.

Coat a sauce pan with cooking spray and place over medium-low heat. Add the egg whites and turmeric. Scramble until well-cooked. (The eggs should look like yellow-orange crumbles.) Next, using a wooden spoon, add the squash, taking care not to break the "noodles." Increase the heat to medium and stir-fry the mixture for 5 to 10 minutes, until the ingredients are well-combined.

YIELD: Makes 6 servings.

NUTRITIONAL ANALYSIS

Per Serving: 149 Calories; 10g Fat (1 g saturated fat); 6g Protein; 10g Carbohydrate; 2g Dietary Fiber; 0mg Cholesterol; 39mg Sodium.

Lime Fish Kebabs°◎

Lime and its juice help keep the bad bacteria at bay, making it a useful, not just flavorful, addition to help with flatulence and general indigestion. Sesame seeds help keep things moving along through the digestive tract, as well as adding a little crunch to your fish.

INGREDIENTS

- Juice of three limes or ¼ cup (60 ml) bottled lime juice
- 2 teaspoons black sesame seeds
- 2 clove garlic, minced
- 1 teaspoon coriander
- 1 teaspoon ground ginger
- 1 teaspoon soy sauce
- 4 wild cod, whitefish, or tilapia filets (about 5 ounces, or 140 g, each), cubed
- 2 zucchini, cut into ¼-inch (6 mm) slices
- 2 yellow squash, cut into ¼-inch (6 mm) slices

In a bowl, combine the lime juice, sesame seeds, garlic, coriander, ginger, and soy sauce. Rub the mixture onto the fish, zucchini, and squash. Place the fish and vegetables on skewers. Place them into a pan with sides (to prevent dripping). Place the pan in the refrigerator, allowing the flavors to marinate at least an hour.

Preheat a grill or the oven to 350 º F (180°C, gas mark 4). Place the skewers on the grill and cook, turning the skewers every few minutes, until the fish turns white. (The amount of time depends upon the cooking method.) If you're baking the fish in the oven and wish to have a "grilled" look, once the fish is almost cooked (still translucent in the center and soft), broil the skewers for about 3 minutes, rotating them every minute. (Be careful to avoid overcooking the fish.)

YIELD: Makes 4 servings.

NUTRITIONAL ANALYSIS
Per Serving: 43 Calories; 1g Fat (trace saturated fat); 2g Protein; 8g Carbohydrate; 3g Dietary Fiber; 0mg Cholesterol; 91 mg Sodium.

"I ate it right off the stick. It would make a great appetizer, too"

—Alissa

● Loose Stools & Diarrhea ○ Fiber ◉ Motility and Lubrication ◎ Indigestion ◉ Really Bad Days

Spinach-Salmon ○◉◉ *(constipation)*

Sautéed Opo squash and layers of spinach replace traditional noodles in this lasagna. What's more, a serving of this lasagna provides a daily dose of those essential fatty acids. You could take a medicine, or you could let your food help you give your body what it needs.

INGREDIENTS

- 1 bag (16 ounces, or 455 g) frozen spinach, thawed and stems removed, or fresh spinach, stems removed
- 1 large Opo squash or other squash, peeled and cut lengthwise into $1/2$-inch (1.25-cm) thick slices
- 1 can (7 ounces, or 200 g) wild salmon or 6 ounces (170 g) wild salmon, cooked medium-rare (see note)
- 2 cups (520 g) Omega 3 Pesto (page 127)

NOTES

This can also be refrigerated and served cold.

Sockeye (red) salmon remains only wild (never farmed); other types of salmon should denote "wild."

"This is a perfect summer replacement for traditional lasagna. It's light and quite attractive. I'd serve this at a brunch or summer dinner party."

—Stephanie

Preheat the oven to 300 º F (150°C, gas mark 2). Coat a $9^{1}/_2$-inch (22.5-cm) oval baking dish with cooking spray.

Press the spinach against the base of a strainer to remove all liquid. Coat a sauté pan with cooking spray and heat on medium. Lay the squash out on the pan, with each piece flat against the pan not overlapping. Lightly sauté the squash, until it turns translucent and the edges brown. Flip over once or twice for even cooking. Remove the squash from the heat and place it on a flat plate to cool. (Do not layer pieces on top of each other.)

Lay the squash in a vertical row down the center of the prepared baking dish, covering the entire length of the pan. (The pieces may overlap, and there will be room on the sides.) Next, unravel half the spinach leaves and arrange them in a layer atop the squash. Layer the salmon on top. Place the other half of spinach over the salmon. Bake for approximately 5 minutes, until the lasagna is warm, but the top layer of spinach isn't dried out or burned.

Remove the lasagna from the oven. Spread the pesto across the top of the spinach. Cut once lengthwise and 6 times width-wise to make 12 servings. Serve warm.

YIELD: Makes 12 servings.

NUTRITIONAL ANALYSIS
Per Serving: 169 Calories; 14g Fat (1 g saturated fat); 9g Protein; 4g Carbohydrate; 2g Dietary Fiber; 9mg Cholesterol; 164mg Sodium.

Stir-Fried Scallops and Sweet Potatoes ⊙◎

In terms of animal products, scallops rank very low on saturated fat and cholesterol content. Paired here with snow pea pods, shitake mushrooms, and sweet potato, this colorful medley is rich in desirable nutrients. The use of kudzu as a thickener helps soothe the stomach and intestines, making this an excellent replacement thickener for people with digestive complaints.

INGREDIENTS

- 3 teaspoons kudzu, crushed (see note)
- 2 tablespoons (28 ml) grapeseed oil, divided
- 1 large or 3 small sweet potatoes, peeled and cut into ½-inch (1.25-cm) slices
- 1 medium red pepper, seeded and cut into squares
- 5 shitake mushrooms, cleaned and halved (see note)
- ½ teaspoon peeled, minced fresh ginger
- 10 snow pea pods, washed, dried, and trimmed
- 1 pound (455 g) sea scallops, halved if very large
- ½ cup (120 ml) low-sodium vegetable broth, heated
- ½ cup (120 ml) light coconut milk
- 2 tablespoons (28 ml) dark agave nectar
- Peel from 1 lime

In a mixing bowl, prepare the kudzu according to the package directions (dissolve it in cold water) and set aside.

In a wok or deep sauté pan, heat 1 tablespoon (14 ml) of the oil. Add the sweet potatoes and stir-fry for 1 minute. Add the pepper and continue stir-frying for another 1 to 2 minutes, until the vegetables are crisp and colorful, but softened. Add the mushrooms, ginger to taste, and snow peas and cook quickly to retain freshness and color. If you're using a sauté pan, remove the vegetable mixture from the pan and set aside. If you're using a wok, push the vegetable mixture to the side of the pan. Add the remaining 1 tablespoon (14 ml) of oil to the wok or pan and cook the scallops, until they become white (versus translucent) and slightly browned.

Add the broth to the kudzu in the mixing bowl, stirring with a whisk so there are no lumps. Add the milk, agave, and lime peel. Pour the mixture into the pan or wok, stirring to combine with the scallops and vegetables. Stir gently and serve warm.

"My favorite dish—a perfect ten for color, texture, and taste!"

—Susan

YIELD: Makes 4 servings.

NUTRITIONAL ANALYSIS

Per Serving: 356 Calories; 15g Fat (7 g saturated fat); 22g Protein; 34g Carbohydrate; 4g Dietary Fiber; 37mg Cholesterol; 204mg Sodium.

NOTES

You can substitute dried mushrooms instead. To prepare them, soak them in water for 20 minutes, drain, and slice.

You can buy kudzu in health food stores and Asian markets.

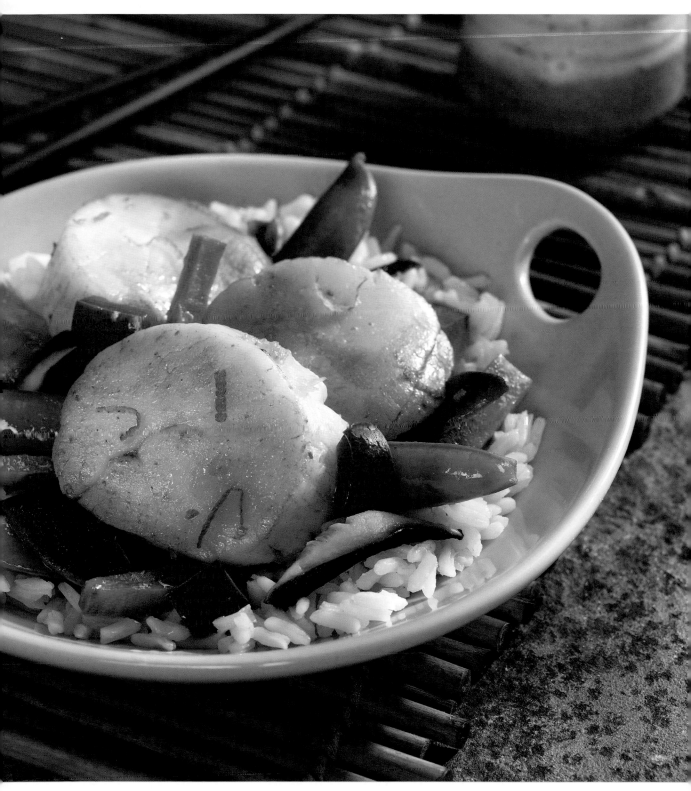

Build-Your-Own Fish Tacos ⦿

your way: fish, tortilla, and steamed or sautéed carrots

◉ *skip the cheese*

This crowd pleaser allows you to build it your way, while they do it their way—a perfect compromise.

INGREDIENTS

- 3 pounds (1.5 kg) fresh, wild caught white fish, cubed, or frozen fish, thawed (see note)
- ¹/₂ cup (120 ml) tangerine juice
- ³/₄ cup (175 ml) lime juice
- 3 teaspoons crushed red pepper
- 3 teaspoons oregano
- 3 teaspoons lemon pepper
- 3 carrots, shredded
- 3 zucchini, shredded
- 2 ounces (55 g) goat cheese or sheep's milk cheese, cubed, such as Manchego cheese
- 10 wheat-free (9-inch, or 22.5-cm) tortillas
- 1 cup (260 g) Tri-Color Salsa (page 126)

In a small bowl, combine the tangerine juice, lime juice, red pepper, oregano, and lemon pepper.

In an 13- by 9-inch (32.5- by 22.5-cm) oven-safe casserole dish, combine the fish and the marinade. Refrigerate for 2 hours, tossing once.

Preheat the oven to 250°F (120°C, gas mark ¹/₂).

In a serving bowl, toss together the carrots and zucchini. Place the cheese in a separate bowl. Place the salsa in a separate bowl.

Bake the tortillas for about 3 minutes, until warm. (If you'd like, you can sprinkle a few drops of water on them first to prevent them from becoming dry.)

Remove the fish from the marinade and discard the marinade. In a sauté pan, stir-fry the fish over medium-low heat, remove from heat, and drain excess water. Serve the fish in the fry pan with the carrots and zucchini, cheese, Tri-Color Salsa, and tortillas around the skillet.

YIELD: Makes 10 servings.

NUTRITIONAL ANALYSIS

Per Serving: 509 Calories; 18g Fat (4 g saturated fat); 36g Protein; 50g Carbohydrate; 5g Dietary Fiber; 88mg Cholesterol; 552mg Sodium.

"I did one with cheese and one without; then I had some stuff without a tortilla. What a great, light meal."

—Brenna

NOTES

If using frozen fish, remove it from the freezer the night before and place in the refrigerator in a container to prevent fluid from leaking into the refrigerator.

You can stir-fry the carrots and zucchini first if you like.

● Loose Stools & Diarrhea ◐ Fiber ◉ Motility and Lubrication ◎ Indigestion ◉ Really Bad Days

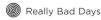

Fish 'n Chips

for diarrhea really bad day, modify Veggie Chips (page 122)

I used frozen, wild fish fillets from Trader Joe's when I made this dish for my tasters. I take great pleasure in going to the fish market for a fresh catch, but I take equally great pleasure in preparing something delicious, healthy, and convenient, using what is in my freezer. Using frozen fish makes this recipe an easy, anytime solution for a digestively friendly and satisfying meal.

INGREDIENTS

- Juice of three limes or 1/4 cup (60 ml) bottled lime juice
- 2 cloves garlic, minced
- 1 teaspoon ground ginger
- 1 teaspoon low-sodium soy sauce
- 1 teaspoon coriander
- 4 wild fish filets, 5 ounces, or 140 g, each (See "Resources" on page 180)
- 4 pieces 6-inch (15-cm) square or 6- by 8-inch (15- by 20-cm) rectangle parchment paper
- 2/3 recipe Veggie Chips (page 122)

Preheat the oven to 425° F (220°C, gas mark 7).

In a shallow mixing bowl or dish, combine the lime juice, garlic, ginger, soy sauce, and coriander. Place the fish in the sauce and marinate in the refrigerator for at least 30 minutes, tossing to coat both sides of the fish.

Remove the fish from the marinade and discard the marinade. Place each piece of fish on the lower half of a piece of parchment paper. Fold the paper over and twist each side to secure the paper wrap. Place the packets on a baking sheet and bake for 8 to 12 minutes, depending on the thickness of the fish. Remove the packets from the oven, place them on individual plates, and unwrap the paper to show fish. Add a side of Veggie Chips and serve.

YIELD: Makes 4 servings.

NUTRITIONAL ANALYSIS

Per Serving: 73 Calories; trace Fat (trace saturated fat); 4g Protein; 16g Carbohydrate; 5g Dietary Fiber; 0mg Cholesterol; 464mg Sodium.

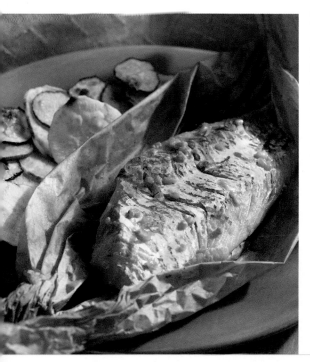

"This isn't the greasy treat I grab in England, which I love, but my stomach hates. But this fish is really moist and flavorful, and I love the colorful crisp chips"

—Matt

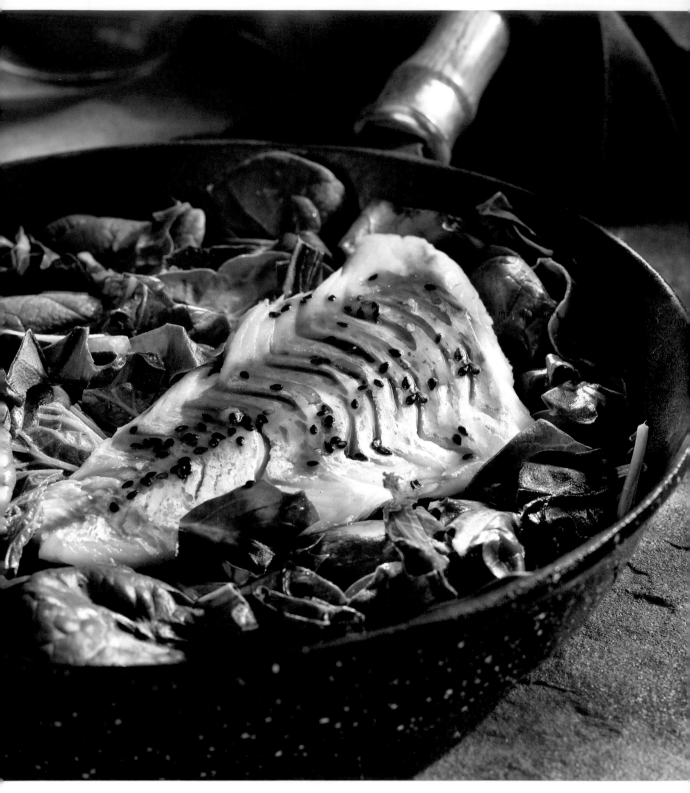

● Loose Stools & Diarrhea ◯ Fiber ◉ Motility and Lubrication ◉ Indigestion ◉ Really Bad Days

Sesame-Ginger Fish and Greens

(constipation)

*This tangy sauce just may be the enabler you've been look-
ing for to get you and your family to eat more greens.*

INGREDIENTS

- $1/2$ cup (120 ml) sesame oil
- $1/4$ cup (60 ml) brown rice vinegar
- 1 tablespoon (14 ml) brown rice syrup
- 2 tablespoons (28 ml) low-sodium soy sauce
- $1/4$ cup (25 g) fresh minced ginger or 3 teaspoons ginger puree
- $1/3$ cup (50 g) black sesame seeds
- 1 tablespoon (14 ml) canola oil
- 8 ounces (225 g) bag mixed greens (kale, chard, mustard greens)
- 4 fillets of wild cod, 5 ounces, or 140 g, each, fresh or frozen (See "Resources" on page 180)

*"Lots of flavor, tangy, fresh, light—
I loved it!"*

—Michael

In a bowl, whisk together the sesame oil, vinegar, rice syrup, soy sauce, ginger, and sesame seeds.

In a sauté pan, place the canola oil or broth over low heat. Add the greens and fish and cook, covered, for about 4 minutes. Turn the fish over, stir in the sauce, and continue to cook for another 2 to 3 minutes, until the fish is white inside and no longer translucent. Remove from the heat.

YIELD: Makes 4 servings.

NUTRITIONAL ANALYSIS
Per Serving: 492 Calories; 38g Fat (5 g saturated fat); 29g Protein; 11g Carbohydrate; 3g Dietary Fiber; 61 mg Cholesterol; 393mg Sodium.

Mediterranean Meat Loaf °

Savory and light, this loaf is bound to be a household favorite. The healing properties of spinach, oats, and carrots combine to help encourage motility and moistness in the digestive tract, which is a desirable effect for combating constipation and promoting digestive health.

INGREDIENTS

- 1 clove garlic, chopped
- 1 small onion, chopped
- 2 tablespoons (28 ml) olive oil
- 1 package (16 ounces, or 455 g) frozen spinach, thawed and drained
- 1 cup (150 g) crumbled sheep's milk feta cheese
- 6 large carrots, julienned
- 1/2 cup (55 g) chopped sun-dried tomatoes, in olive oil or 4 ounces (115 g) tomato tapenade from a jar
- 1 1/2 pounds (680 g) ground turkey breast
- 1 cup (155 g) rolled oats

Preheat the oven to 400° F (200°C, gas mark 6). Lightly coat a loaf pan with cooking spray.

In a sauté pan, sauté the garlic and onions in olive oil over low heat, until soft but not brown. Stir in the spinach and cook for 2 to 3 minutes. Remove the spinach mixture from the heat and cool completely. Stir in the cheese.

Spray another sauté pan with cooking spray and sauté the carrots until soft. (Or microwave them in a microwave-safe bowl on high power.)

In a large bowl, mix the tomatoes, turkey, and oats. Press two-thirds of the turkey mixture into the prepared pan. Layer the carrots on top of the turkey mixture, and then layer the spinach mixture on top of the carrots. Cover with rest of the turkey mixture. Bake for 30 to 35 minutes, cool for 5 to 10 minutes, then place onto a serving plate, slice, and serve.

YIELD: Makes 6 servings.

NUTRITIONAL ANALYSIS
Per Serving: 403 Calories; 22g Fat (7 g saturated fat); 29g Protein; 24g Carbohydrate; 7g Dietary Fiber; 112mg Cholesterol; 492mg Sodium.

"I can't wait to have this again"

—Rosie

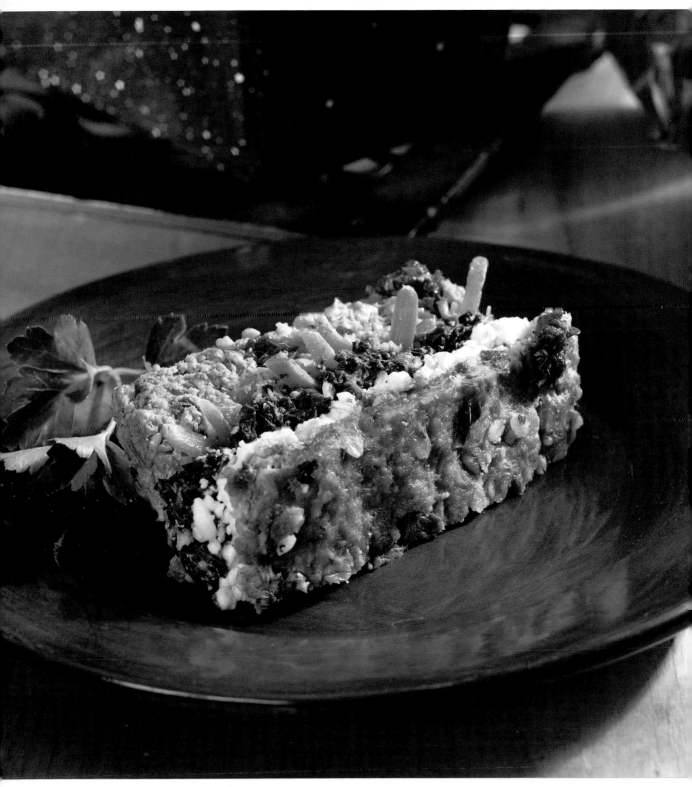

Turkey Meatballs© *try sesame or olive oil*

● *add cayenne pepper, exchange onion for button mushroom, and exchange buckwheat for oat groats*

These little meatballs can stand alone with some greens, jump into your favorite sauce, or stand alone as a snack or appetizer. So versatile, these can be made and frozen to have on hand for different occasions.

INGREDIENTS

- ½ cup (80 g) chopped onion
- 1 clove elephant garlic, minced
- 1 tablespoon (14 ml) olive oil
- 1 pound (455 g) lean ground turkey breast
- 3 tablespoons (45 ml) liquid egg whites
- ½ cup (85 g) oat groats
- 2 tablespoons (10 g) grated Parmesan cheese
- 3 teaspoons tomato paste
- 3 teaspoons basil
- 3 teaspoons oregano
- Salt (optional)

In a sauté pan, sauté the onion and garlic in the oil and set them aside to cool.

In a mixing bowl, combine the turkey, egg whites, oats, cheese, tomato paste, basil, oregano, and salt, if using. Add the garlic and onion. Using your hands, pinch off some mixture to form a ball. (The smaller the balls, the faster they'll cook.)

In a large sauté pan, sauté the meatballs about 6 to 8 minutes, until golden brown and cooked thoroughly. (There should not be any pink meat on the inside.)

YIELD: Makes 10 servings.

NUTRITIONAL ANALYSIS

Per Serving: 174 Calories; 6g Fat (2 g saturated fat); 13g Protein; 18g Carbohydrate; 2g Dietary Fiber; 3 7mg Cholesterol; 88 mg Sodium.

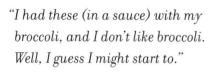

"I had these (in a sauce) with my broccoli, and I don't like broccoli. Well, I guess I might start to."

—Michael

NOTE

Instead of sautéing the meatballs, you could bake them in a 375º F oven (190°C, gas mark 5) in muffin pans coated with cooking spray, for about 10 minutes.

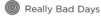

"Jerk" Turkey Burgers

The combination of spices and lime juice here are sure to make any unwanted critters in your digestive tract run for the exit sign. Why not try Papaya Soup (page 79) before a burger for optimal digestion?

INGREDIENTS

- 1 teaspoon thyme
- 1 teaspoon fennel seeds
- 1 teaspoon ground ginger
- 1 teaspoon allspice
- 1 teaspoon turmeric
- 1 teaspoon paprika
- 1 teaspoon marjoram
- ¼ cup (60 ml) lime juice
- 2 tablespoons (28 ml) light soy sauce
- 3 teaspoons brown mustard
- 1 tablespoon (14 ml) dark agave nectar
- 1 pound (455 g) lean ground turkey breast
- 1 cup (160 g) diced onion
- 2 cloves garlic, minced

In a large mixing bowl, whisk together the thyme, fennel, ginger, allspice, turmeric, paprika, marjoram, lime juice, soy sauce, mustard, and agave until all the ingredients dissolve together. Add the turkey and mix to combine thoroughly. Place the turkey mixture in a glass container with a cover. Refrigerator to marinate for at least 2 to 4 hours (ideally overnight).

Coat a sauté pan with cooking spray and sauté the onion and garlic over low heat until soft and golden brown. Fold the onion and garlic into turkey mixture. Using your hands, make 30 to 40 gum ball–size or 10 to 15 golf ball–size patties.

Lightly coat a heavy skillet with cooking spray and heat it over medium-low heat. Cook the turkey patties on each side for 3 to 5 minutes, until golden cooked all the way through. (Be careful not to cook with too much heat as the burgers will turn golden before the meat is cooked.)

YIELD: Makes 15 servings.

NUTRITIONAL ANALYSIS
Per Serving: 60 Calories; 3g Fat (1 g saturated fat); 6g Protein; 3g Carbohydrate; trace Dietary Fiber; 24mg Cholesterol; 180mg Sodium.

"This is a backyard BBQ must-have!"

—Jon

Turkey Wraps ●◉◉ *(constipation and diarrhea) add greens for constipation*

Easy and fast, these wraps make a quick breakfast, a portable lunch, or a satisfying snack. Eat them on the spot or roll 'em, wrap 'em (in plastic wrap or wax paper), and grab 'em to go.

INGREDIENTS

- 6 slices low or no-sodium, hormone-free turkey breast (I use Applegate Farms.)
- 1 cup Timeless Tapenade (page 129), No Más Gas Guacamole (page 137), Prune-Ginger Chutney (page 128), Pineapple Chutney (page 127), or your favorite spread
- ½ recipe Brightly Sautéed Greens (page 117) (optional)

On a flat surface, lay the turkey slices flat. Spread a thin layer of Timeless Tapenade, No Más Gas Guacamole, Prune-Ginger Chutney, Pineapple Chutney, or your favorite spread on each slice. Top it with Brightly Sautéed Greens, if using. Roll each slice up or fold in half.

YIELD: Makes 2 servings.

NUTRITIONAL ANALYSIS
Per Serving: 257 Calories; 16g Fat (2 g saturated fat); 18g Protein; 12g Carbohydrate; 5g Dietary Fiber; 26mg Cholesterol; 1178mg Sodium.

> *"I had those turkey wraps again today. They're such a great snack."*
>
> —David

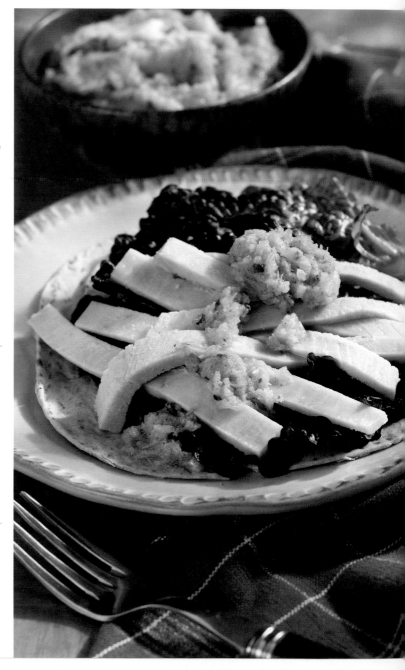

Chicken Bouillabaisse ⊙◎◉ *(constipation)*

Saffron excels as a digestive aid to help restore natural balance and calm throughout the digestive system. Just a pinch is all you need to reap the benefits of this prized spice. Citrus peel enhances digestion by helping to alleviate constipation.

INGREDIENTS

- 1 bulb fennel, cored and sliced
- 2 cloves garlic, minced
- 1½ cups (355 ml) low-sodium chicken broth
- 1 pound (455 g) boneless, skinless chicken breast, cut into 16 equal pieces
- 2 cups (200 g) chopped okra
- 1 tablespoon (14 ml) white wine or apple cider vinegar
- ½ cup (120 ml) water
- ⅛ teaspoon saffron
- Peel of ½ orange

Preheat the oven to 325º F (170°C, gas mark 3.)

In a large iron paella or deep oven-safe saucepan with a lid, sauté the garlic and fennel in 1 cup of the broth until tender but not brown. Drain off the juice and reserve it for basting later. Add the chicken to the paella or saucepan, spreading the fennel around them and sauté in the remaining broth on medium heat, until brown. Cover and cook 10 minutes, flipping the chicken over once. Cover the chicken with the okra and cook briefly on high heat, then reduce the heat to medium heat. Add the vinegar, water, saffron, and orange peel and transfer to the oven. Bake for 20 to 25 minutes, basting a few times with the reserved juice.

"Tastes rich — is it?"

–Karla

YIELD: Makes 6 servings.

NUTRITIONAL ANALYSIS

Per Serving: 124 Calories; 3g Fat (1 g saturated fat); 21g Protein; 6g Carbohydrate; 2g Dietary Fiber; 46mg Cholesterol; 74mg Sodium.

NOTE

Fennel is also called anise.

Root Vegetable-Chicken-Apple Sausage Stew °

● use string beans instead of greens   ◉ (diarrhea) use string beans instead of greens

Mary Ross's quote says it best (see below). Whether seeking physical or emotional comfort, this lightly sweet, colorful, soft stew gives you nutrients and a bit of warm TLC.

INGREDIENTS

- 1 butternut or acorn squash
- 2 small sweet potatoes, peeled and cut into pieces
- 1½ cups low-sodium vegetable broth or chicken broth or grapeseed oil, divided
- 2 cups (140 g) kale, spinach, chard, or collards, washed, chopped, and stems removed
- 4 chicken-apple sausages, fully cooked and sliced, such as Applegate Farms
- Cayenne pepper
- Dried thyme, crushed

Preheat the oven to 400° F (200°C, gas mark 6).

Pierce squash with the point of a knife and microwave on high power for 3 to 4 minutes. When the squash is cool enough to handle, peel, seed, and cube it.

In a sauté pan, sauté the squash and sweet potatoes in ½ cup (120 ml) of the broth or grapeseed oil, until they begin to soften. Add the greens, continuing to sauté, stirring frequently. Stir in the remaining broth, then add the sausages and pepper and thyme to taste. Bake for 30 minutes, basting 2 or 3 times with the pan juices. Serve hot.

YIELD: Makes 8 servings.

NUTRITIONAL ANALYSIS
Per Serving: 168 Calories; 1g Fat (trace saturated fat); 7g Protein; 36g Carbohydrate; 5g Dietary Fiber; 16mg Cholesterol; 148mg Sodium.

"This takes comfort food to a whole new level."

—Mary Ross

NOTE

Instead of sautéing the vegetables, you could place all of the vegetables in a baking pan and drizzle with olive oil. Roast in a 450°F (230°C, gas mark 8) oven for 30 to 45 minutes, until the vegetables begin to cook.

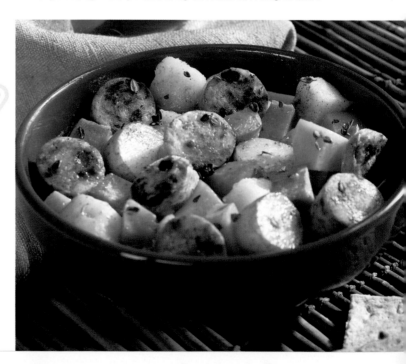

Fig-Chicken Curry ◉◉◉ *(constipation) over spinach*

This curry pairs figs and fenugreek for flavor and substance. Additionally, both have long histories as natural laxatives.

INGREDIENTS

- 1¹/₂ pounds (700 g) halved fresh figs (see note)
- 1 teaspoon ground fenugreek seeds
- 1 cup (235 ml) light coconut milk
- 24 ounces (670 g) boneless, skinless chicken breasts, cubed

Preheat the oven to 400° F (200°C, gas mark 6).

In a food processor, puree the figs, fenugreek seeds, and milk.

Place the chicken in a 9-inch (22.5-cm) square baking dish and pour the fig mixture over the chicken. Bake for 25 to 30 minutes, until the chicken is fully cooked. (Don't overcook the chicken, It should be tender.)

YIELD: Makes 4 servings.

NUTRITIONAL ANALYSIS
Per Serving: 466 Calories; 19g Fat (14 g saturated fat); 41 g Protein; 36g Carbohydrate; 7g Dietary Fiber; 104mg Cholesterol; 101 mg Sodium.

"I love how sweet and creamy this dish tasted."

—Becca

NOTES

You may substitute dried figs. Soak them in water for 1 hour to reconstitute, drain, and slice in half.

This dish is great tossed over soba noodles, steamed spinach, or steamed cauliflower and broccoli.

Wheat-Free Chickensadillas

These are a more traditional version of quesadillas than the Chicken Greensadillas (recipe on right) and a crowd favorite. Try out different tortillas to see what flavor combination you like best. This is likely to be a family favorite.

INGREDIENTS

- 1 (6 ounces, or 170 g) grilled chicken breast
- 2 teaspoons extra virgin olive oil
- 2 ounces (55 g) sheep's milk feta cheese, crumbled
- 1 jarred roasted red pepper
- 4 (7-inch, or 17.5-cm) wheat-free tortillas

Preheat the oven to 325º F (170°C, gas mark 3). Lightly coat a baking sheet with cooking spray.

In a food processor, blend the chicken, oil, cheese, and pepper, until the mixture no longer contains any chunks of chicken or pepper. Spread the mixture evenly across the center of each tortilla; then fold the tortillas in half. Bake for 10 to 15 minutes, until the edges appear crisp. Remove from the heat and cut each tortilla in half again.

YIELD: Makes 4 servings.

NUTRITIONAL ANALYSIS
Per Serving: 362 Calories; 13g Fat (4 g saturated fat); 19g Protein; 41g Carbohydrate; 3g Dietary Fiber; 42mg Cholesterol; 527mg Sodium.

"Bob ate them all. Really. I don't think anyone else got any. They are his favorite."

—Edna

NOTES

I use herb-roasted chicken breast from my grocery's prepared food section.

Try Healthy Hemp from French Meadow Bakery or make Buck-the-Wheat Tortillas, (page 119).

● Loose Stools & Diarrhea　◐ Fiber　◉ Motility and Lubrication　◎ Indigestion　◉ Really Bad Days

 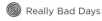

Chicken Greensadillas°

Passing on a grain tortilla, this light snack or meal helps get in the greens in a colorful and tasty way.

INGREDIENTS

- 1 bunch collard greens (approximately 12 leaves)
- 1 (6 ounces, or 170 g) grilled chicken breast (see note)
- 1 jarred whole roasted red pepper
- 2 ounces (55 g) sheep's milk feta cheese, crumbled (optional)
- 2 teaspoons extra virgin olive oil

NOTE

I use herb-roasted chicken breast from my grocery's prepared food section.

Preheat the oven to 325° F (170°C, gas mark 3). Lightly coat two large baking sheets with cooking spray.

Wash the collards well. Using a scissors, cut along the entire stem of the leaf to separate each leaf in half to make about 24 halves. Prepare a steamer pot; place the collards into the steamer and lightly steam, until the collards turn bright green but are not truly wilted. Immediately remove the collards from the steamer and lay out on a flat surface to cool.

In a food processor, combine the chicken, pepper, cheese, and oil into a thick mixture, until the mixture no longer contains any chunks of chicken or pepper.

Arrange the collard leaves vertically on a flat surface. Use two spoons to drop a spoonful of filling into the center of a collard leaf half. Fold each leaf in half and gently press on the filling to spread it out from the center almost to the edge. (Don't press too hard or the filling will come out of the sides.) Place each of the filled greens, not touching, on the prepared baking sheet. Bake for 10 to 15 minutes, until the edges of the greens turn a bit darker but not burnt. Serve warm.

YIELD: Makes 6 servings.

NUTRITIONAL ANALYSIS
Per Serving: 87 Calories; 5g Fat (2 g saturated fat); 8g Protein; 1g Carbohydrate; trace Dietary Fiber; 28mg Cholesterol; 123mg Sodium.

"This seems like the perfect afternoon snack—fun, tasty, and easy to eat."

—Andrea

Chicken-Mushroom Risotto ⊚

omit spinach and parmesan; use scallion bulb instead of onions and shallots

(diarrhea) omit spinach and parmesan; use scallion bulb instead of onions and shallots

The different types of mushrooms offer numerous health benefits, including stimulation of the immune system. Mushrooms should be eaten cooked, which is not difficult to accomplish as they imbue dishes with a range of flavors from mild to strong. Play around with a combination of mushrooms or stick with just one. Enjoy what mushrooms do for your meal, as well as for your health!

INGREDIENTS

- 2 tablespoons (28 ml) olive oil or canola oil, divided
- 1 clove garlic, minced
- ³/₄ cup (120 g) diced shallots or sweet onion
- ¹/₂ delicata or butternut squash, peeled and cubed
- ¹/₃ cup (20 g) sliced shiitake mushrooms
- ¹/₃ cup (20 g) sliced enoki mushrooms
- ¹/₃ cup (20 g) chanterelle mushrooms
- 4 chicken thighs or 2 chicken breasts (6 ounces, or 170 g, each), cut into cubes
- 32 ounces (896 ml) low-sodium chicken broth or vegetable broth
- 1¹/₂ cups (335 g) Arborio rice
- ¹/₂ cup (15 g) fresh spinach leaves, stems removed (optional)
- 3 tablespoons (45 ml) balsamic vinegar
- ¹/₂ cup (50 g) Parmesan cheese (optional)

In a sauté pan, heat 1 tablespoon of the oil over medium heat. Sauté the garlic, shallots or onion, and squash until slightly browned. Add the mushrooms and continue to sauté for a minute or two. Remove the vegetables from the sauté pan and reserve.

Coat the sauté pan with cooking spray and add the chicken. Cook for 3 to 5 minutes, until the chicken is no longer raw, but not dry. Remove the chicken from pan and set aside with the vegetables.

In a saucepan, heat the broth over medium heat.

In the saucepan where the vegetables were cooked, heat the remaining 1 tablespoon (14 ml) oil, and toss the rice in the oil, until it is coated. Pour in 1 cup of the hot broth and stir the rice, continuously adding broth and stirring for about 20 minutes. (You need to watch it at this point so it doesn't burn.) When the rice is al dente, not soft, turn down the heat and fold back in the vegetables and chicken pieces. Add the spinach, if using. (It will wilt on contact.) Scoop the risotto into individual serving plates and pour a spoonful of the vinegar over each portion. Pass the cheese, if using, in a small bowl.

"The rice is crunchy, which is good for me. I don't like soft pastas or mushy foods."

—Aaron

YIELD: Makes 6 servings.

NUTRITIONAL ANALYSIS
Per Serving: 457 Calories; 18g Fat (5 g saturated fat); 26g Protein; 55g Carbohydrate; 2g Dietary Fiber; 58 mg Cholesterol; 211 mg Sodium.

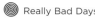

Raspberry Chicken ●◎

exchange blackberries for raspberries and use canola oil in place of mustard

Full of fiber and other nutrients, raspberries are at once both sweet and sour; they form the backbone of this tangy chicken dish.

INGREDIENTS

- 3 cups (750 g) frozen raspberries, thawed and pureed
- 1 cup (235 ml) unsweetened raspberry juice
- ⅓ cup (75 ml) balsamic vinegar
- 1 tablespoon (14 ml) low-sodium soy sauce
- 2 tablespoons (30 g) Homestyle Mustard (page 138) or prepared Dijon mustard
- 1 bunch fresh basil leaves, set aside 6 leaves for garnish, remove stems and chop the rest
- 3 boneless, skinless chicken breasts, 6 ounces (170 g) each
- 2 teaspoons canola or grapeseed oil

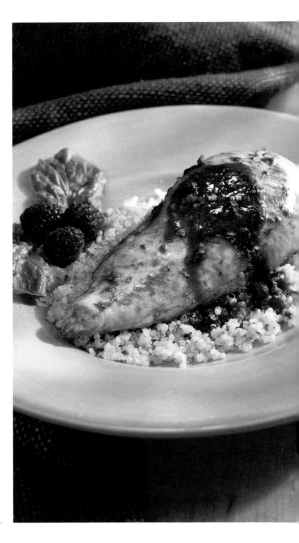

In a bowl, combine the raspberries, raspberry juice, vinegar, soy sauce, mustard, and chopped basil. Divide the mixture in half.

In a flat, glass pan big enough to lay the chicken flat and not touching, put half of the mixture. Add the chicken. Marinate for 1 hour in the refrigerator, spooning the sauce over the chicken once or twice. Drain off the marinade.

In a skillet, heat the oil over medium heat. Add the chicken and cook for 2 minutes on each side. Slice the chicken on an angle, place it on serving plate or individual plates, and spoon the sauce from the pan over the slices. Garnish with the reserved basil leaves.

YIELD: Makes 4 servings.

NUTRITIONAL ANALYSIS
Per Serving: 458 Calories; 8g Fat (1 g saturated fat); 41g Protein; 58g Carbohydrate; 8g Dietary Fiber; 108mg Cholesterol; 347mg Sodium.

Buffalo Chili°◉

Coriander is known as a digestive aid. (In fact, some healthcare practitioners recommend using it as a digestif, mixing ½ teaspoon crushed coriander seeds into 1 cup (235 ml) hot water and drinking it 30 minutes before meals.) Here coriander enhances the flavor of buffalo meat, which is lower in saturated fat than beef.

INGREDIENTS

- ¼ cup (60 ml) canola oil
- 1 small red onion or ½ sweet onion, diced
- 3 medium carrots, peeled and cut into ½-inch (1.25-cm) slices
- 2 small yellow squash, scrubbed and cut into ½-inch (1.25-cm) slices
- 2 small zucchini, scrubbed and diced
- 1 teaspoon dried or fresh coriander
- 1 tablespoon dried chili powder
- 1 teaspoon cumin
- ½ teaspoon cayenne pepper or paprika (optional)
- 1½ pounds (700 g) ground buffalo meat
- 2 cans (14½ ounces, or 400 g, each) or 1 can (28 ounces, or 784 g) fire-roasted tomatoes, chopped
- 3 cups (780 g) mild or medium salsa

In a deep sauce pot, heat the oil over medium heat. Sauté the onion, then add the carrots, squash, and zucchini, stirring often, until the edges are brown but the vegetables are not soft. Toss some of the coriander, chili powder, cumin and cayenne or paprika, if using, into the vegetables as you cook them so the flavor of the spices adheres to them. Transfer the vegetables to a medium bowl and set aside.

Add the buffalo meat to the skillet and cook on medium heat, stirring often, to brown. (If the meat sticks to the pan, add a little of canola oil to the center of the pan, heat it up, and then continue sautéing the buffalo meat.) Stir in the rest of the coriander, chili powder, cumin, and cayenne or paprika, if using, to combine them with the buffalo meat. Drain buffalo meat if necessary in a colander. (Since the buffalo is lean, this is often not necessary.) Return the buffalo meat and vegetables to the pot and add the tomatoes in their juice. Pour in the salsa and cook over medium heat for 15 minutes, stirring frequently. Reduce heat to a simmer and cook for 40 minutes. Or you could refrigerate at this point and reheat on low for 20 to 30 minutes, stirring often, before serving.

"Perfect. This belongs at a Super Bowl party."

—Michael

YIELD: Makes 12 servings.

NUTRITIONAL ANALYSIS
Per Serving: 140 Calories; 6g Fat (1 g saturated fat); 14g Protein; 12g Carbohydrate; 4g Dietary Fiber; 26mg Cholesterol; 332mg Sodium.

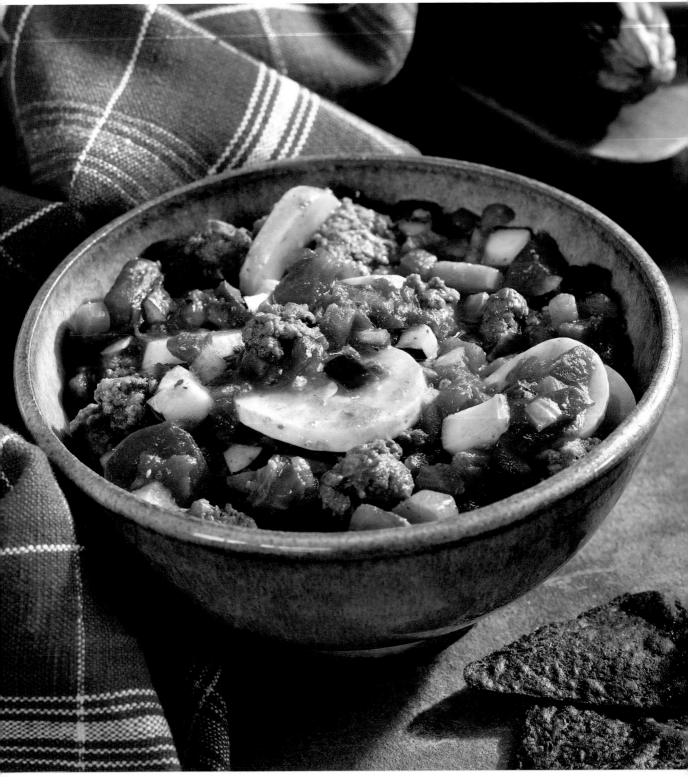

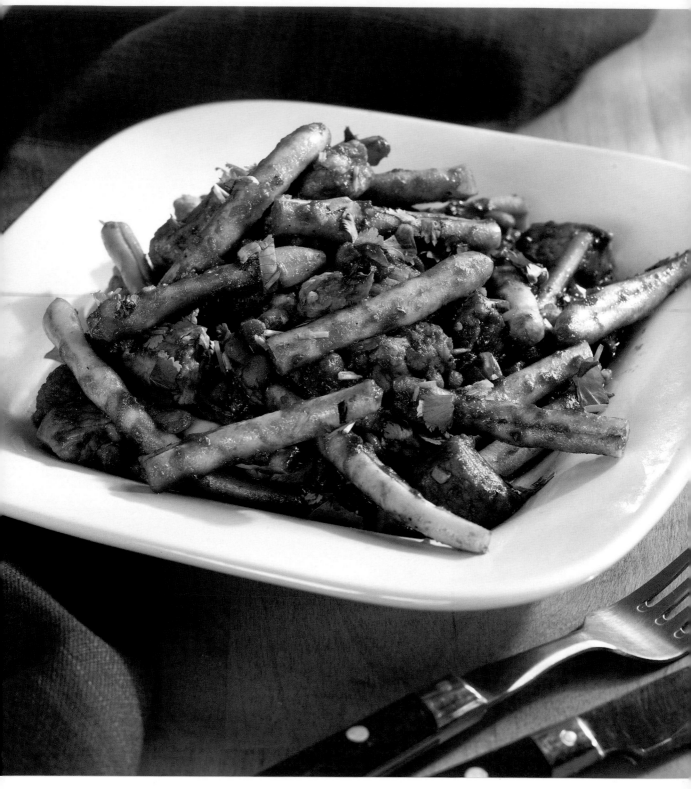

● Loose Stools & Diarrhea ◐ Fiber ◉ Motility and Lubrication ◎ Indigestion ◉ Really Bad Days

Pork-Tendered for Better Digestion°◉

Known to enhance digestion, bitters (such as gentian root) are a known digestif in Europe. In this recipe, bitters impart bitter-sweetness for a surprisingly light, yet lively dish.

INGREDIENTS

- 8 ounces (225 g) lean pork from a tenderloin or thick chops
- 3 cloves garlic, minced
- 3 tablespoons (45 ml) olive oil
- 1 can (14 ounces, or 400 g) fire-roasted tomatoes
- 1/2 cup (130 g) tomato paste
- 2 ounces (60 ml) bitters, such as Angostura
- 1/16 teaspoon salt
- 2 cups (400 g) cooked lentils
- 2 tablespoons (2 g) coarsely chopped cilantro
- 1 1/4 cups (140 g) trimmed and halved green beans

Freeze the pork for about 20 minutes (not longer); remove from freezer and slice thinly.

In a skillet, place the garlic and lightly brown the pork in the oil on medium-low heat. After a few minutes, add the tomatoes, tomato paste, and bitters, stirring frequently. Season with the salt and let simmer for about 10 minutes. (Pork needs to be cooked thoroughly.) Add the lentils to the tomato-pork mixture. Simmer until hot, stir in the cilantro, and taste. (Add additional salt or cilantro if necessary.) In a saucepan, boil the green beans. Drain the green beans. Fold green beans into the stew and serve.

Makes 6 servings.

NUTRITIONAL ANALYSIS

Per Serving: 214 Calories; 9g Fat (1 g saturated fat); 16g Protein; 23g Carbohydrate; 8g Dietary Fiber; 25mg Cholesterol; 223 mg Sodium.

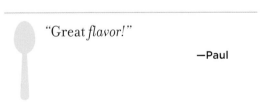

"Great flavor!"

—Paul

CHAPTER 3

The Supporting Cast:
Soups, Salads, Appetizers, and Sides

These recipes can support a Principle (see Chapter 2) for a larger meal, combine with other Supporting Cast recipes for a delicious medley, or take center stage solo for a smaller, digestively beneficial eating occasion.

Peach Soup°◉ *(constipation)*

Peaches benefit the digestive system by encouraging the release of digestive juices, as well as mild laxative properties. Especially cooked, peaches also help reduce inflammation and irritation.

INGREDIENTS

- 7 ripe peaches
- 1 tablespoon (14 ml) lime juice
- 3 tablespoons (45 ml) agave nectar
- 2 tablespoons (28 ml) champagne vinegar or apple cider vinegar instead
- 1 cup (235 ml) water
- 3 whole allspice berries
- Peel of 1 lime

In a large saucepan, cover 6 peaches with boiling water and let stand for 2 minutes. Drain, peel, and remove the pits from the peaches. Discard the water. Place peaches in a food processor and puree.

In the saucepan, bring the peach puree, lime juice, agave, vinegar, water, and allspice to a boil, stirring continuously. Reduce the heat and simmer, continuing to stir, for 10 minutes. Remove the mixture from heat and take out the allspice. Let the mixture cool until the pot is at room temperature. Refrigerate until cold.

Prior to serving the soup, slice the remaining peach. Garnish each serving with a peach slice and some lime peel.

"I love this soup."

—Mel

YIELD: Makes 8 servings.

NUTRITIONAL ANALYSIS
Per Serving: 67 Calories; trace Fat (trace saturated fat); 1g Protein; 18g Carbohydrate; 2g Dietary Fiber; 0mg Cholesterol; 3mg Sodium.

● Loose Stools & Diarrhea ○ Fiber ◉ Motility and Lubrication ◎ Indigestion ◉ Really Bad Days

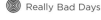

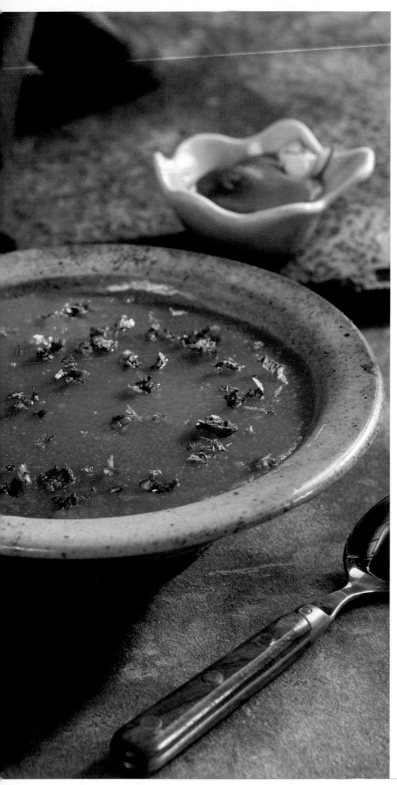

Papaya Soup
(constipation)

Papaya contains a digestive enzyme that helps to break down protein. Start with this chilled soup before eating animal protein, such as a "Jerk" Turkey Burger (page 65) or Devilish Eggs (page 90).

INGREDIENTS

- 10 fresh mint leaves
- 2 papayas, skinned and seeded, or 1 package ($^3/_4$ pound, or 340 g) pre-cut papaya
- 40 almonds or 2 tablespoons (30 g) almond butter
- 2 tablespoons (28 ml) freshly squeezed lime juice

In a food processor, puree the mint leaves and papaya. Transfer the mixture to a metal bowl and refrigerate it to chill.

In the food processor, process the almonds or almond butter and lime juice together. Fold into the papaya mixture or drizzle it on top. Serve the soup cold.

YIELD: Makes 4 servings.

NUTRITIONAL ANALYSIS
Per Serving: 112 Calories; 5g Fat (1 g saturated fat); 2g Protein; 17g Carbohydrate; 3g Dietary Fiber; 0mg Cholesterol; 6mg Sodium.

"This has a light, mild flavor, but it's totally satisfying"

—Amy

Curried Butternut Squash and Apple Soup°°

This sweet soup provides a gentle treat for cool days. Enjoy it with an egg white dish for breakfast or with a handful of nuts for lunch or dinner.

INGREDIENTS

- 3 cups (480 g) chopped onions, divided
- $^2/_3$ cup (85 g) chopped carrots
- $^1/_2$ cup (50 g) chopped celery
- 3 tablespoons (45 ml) olive oil, divided
- 1$^3/_4$ cup (245 g) peeled and diced butternut squash
- 3 cloves garlic, minced
- 2 cups (475 ml) water
- 2 cups (475 ml) vegetable broth
- 3 teaspoons fresh oregano
- 3 tablespoons olive oil
- 1 Granny Smith apple, peeled and diced
- $^1/_2$ tablespoon hot curry powder
- $^1/_2$ tablespoon sweet curry powder
- 1 teaspoon dill weed
- 3 teaspoons cinnamon powder or cinnamon sticks for garnish (optional)

In a large pot, sauté 2 cups (320 g) of the onions with the carrots and celery in 2 tablespoons (28 ml) of the oil over medium heat until the onions are soft but not brown. Add the squash and garlic and continue to sauté for about 5 minutes, until the squash is soft and the garlic is golden brown. Add the water, broth, and oregano. Cover and simmer until all vegetables are soft.

In a skillet, heat the remaining 1 tablespoon (14 ml) oil over low heat and add the remaining cup of onions; sauté until golden brown. Add the apple and continue to sauté for about 3 minutes, until the apple is soft and lightly browned. Add the curry powder and cook for 1 more minute. Remove from the heat and mix in the dill.

In a blender, puree the vegetables in batches. Return the pureed vegetables to the pot and fold in the apple-onion mixture. Simmer for approximately 5 minutes. Garnish with cinnamon or cinnamon sticks, if using.

YIELD: Makes 6 servings.

NUTRITIONAL ANALYSIS

Per Serving: 252 Calories; 15g Fat (2 g saturated fat); 4g Protein; 27g Carbohydrate; 6g Dietary Fiber; 1 mg Cholesterol; 564mg Sodium.

"This is a great adaptation. I really like it."

—Kath

● Loose Stools & Diarrhea ◐ Fiber ◉ Motility and Lubrication ◎ Indigestion ◉ Really Bad Days

Spooner's Chestnut Soup ● ◎ ◉ *(diarrhea)*

I first tried chestnut soup at a friend's holiday gathering. This adaptation replaces dairy for a delicious, easy to digest holiday soup.

INGREDIENTS

- ¹/₄ cup (60 ml) grapeseed oil
- 2 cups (200 g) chopped celery
- 1 sweet onion, chopped
- 3 cups (705 ml) low-sodium vegetable broth
- 1 cup (235 ml) water
- ¹/₄ cup (15 g) chopped fresh parsley
- 1 teaspoon thyme
- 6 fresh basil leaves, diced, divided
- 1 can (15¹/₂ ounces, or 445 g) chestnuts in water, drained
- ¹/₄ cup (30 g) buckwheat flour or chestnut flour
- 2 tablespoons (28 ml) apple cider vinegar
- ¹/₁₆ teaspoon salt
- Black pepper

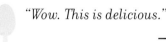

"Wow. This is delicious."

—Barbara

In a large soup pot, heat the oil over low heat and toss in the celery and onion. Cover and cook about 10 minutes, stirring occasionally, until the vegetables soften but are not brown. Stir in the broth, water, parsley, thyme, and half of the basil leaves. Add the chestnuts. Pour in the flour and whisk until there are virtually no clumps. Simmer for 20 minutes. Remove from the heat and let cool for 3 minutes.

In batches, pour the mixture into blender and puree. Return the mixture to the soup pot, add the vinegar, salt, and pepper to taste, and let simmer for at least 5 minutes. Pour into bowls and garnish with the reserved basil.

YIELD: Makes 10 servings.

NUTRITIONAL ANALYSIS
Per Serving: 165 Calories; 7g Fat (1 g saturated fat); 3g Protein; 24g Carbohydrate; 4g Dietary Fiber; 0mg Cholesterol; 55mg Sodium.

Fennel-White Bean Soup ◑◎

Bean soup may sound totally off limits. The addition of fennel and fennel seeds makes the bark of these beans much worse than their bite.

INGREDIENTS

- 1 fennel bulb with $1/4$ inch (6 mm) of the stems (set leaves aside), sliced
- 1 cup (235 ml) broth
- 2 teaspoons fennel seeds
- 1 teaspoon fresh lemon peel, grated
- $1/2$ can (15 ounces, or 430 g) white beans, rinsed and drained

In a large skillet with a cover, place the fennel, broth, fennel seeds, and lemon peel and heat over medium. Cook for about 10 minutes, or until the fennel softens. Reduce the heat to low, add the beans, and simmer for 5 to 10 minutes. Remove from heat and let cool.

Transfer the mixture to a food processor and puree. Serve warm or cold. Garnish with a sprig or two of fennel leaves.

YIELD: Makes 4 servings.

NUTRITIONAL ANALYSIS
Per Serving: 146 Calories; 1g Fat (trace saturated fat); 9g Protein; 28g Carbohydrate; 7g Dietary Fiber; 0mg Cholesterol; 37mg Sodium.

"Don't tell anyone. I always get gas from beans. I didn't get gas from this soup. I swear. Got any other ones?"

—A.W.

NOTE

Fennel is also called anise.

Pumpkin Punch ◎

◉ *very ripe bananas*

● *use less ripe banana (may need to puree)*

Whether cold or hot, this thick soup digests easily and really helps calm an irritated gastrointestinal tract.

INGREDIENTS

- 2 teaspoons canola oil
- $1/4$ cup (25 g) minced fresh ginger
- 3 cups fresh or canned pumpkin, mashed
- 1 medium ripe banana, mashed
- 8 cups (1880 ml) vegetable broth
- $1/16$ teaspoon salt
- Dash powdered allspice
- Fresh mint, chopped (optional)

In a large, deep pot, heat the oil and sauté the ginger over low heat. Add the pumpkin, banana, and broth. Bring the mixture to a boil, cover, reduce the heat, and simmer for 40 minutes.

Transfer the mixture to a blender and puree. Add the salt and allspice. Pour into serving dishes and garnish with the mint, if using.

YIELD: Makes 10 servings.

NUTRITIONAL ANALYSIS
Per Serving: 175 Calories; 4g Fat (1 g saturated fat); 6g Protein; 3 0g Carbohydrate; 5g Dietary Fiber; 2mg Cholesterol; 1318mg Sodium.

"I like it cold, like for breakfast in the summer."

—Anna

● Loose Stools & Diarrhea   ◐ Fiber   ◑ Motility and Lubrication   ◎ Indigestion   ◉ Really Bad Days

Dairy-Free, Oh-So-Tasty Fish Chowder °◎

By substituting almond milk for cow's milk or cream, you get a nutty, light chowder that's soon to be a favorite.

INGREDIENTS

- ¹/₂ cup (45 g) diced fennel
- 2 tablespoons (28 ml) grapeseed oil
- 1 teaspoon thyme
- 2 tablespoons (28 ml) brown rice vinegar
- 3 teaspoons tomato paste
- 2 medium green apples, peeled, cored, and cubed
- 1 cup (235 ml) fish broth or clam juice
- 1 pound (455 g) orange roughy, white fillets, or wild salmon
- 1¹/₂ cups (355 ml) plain almond milk

In an 8-quart (8-L) pot, lightly sauté the fennel in the oil until it softens.

In a small saucepan, add the thyme, vinegar, fennel, and tomato paste. Stir and cook for 3 minutes. Add the apples and broth or clam juice. Bring to a boil, reduce the heat, and simmer for 15 minutes, stirring every 2 or 3 minutes. Add the fish and simmer on low for 5 minutes. Reduce the heat as low as possible before adding the almond milk and stir for a minute to combine. Remove from the heat and serve warm.

YIELD: Makes 4 servings.

NUTRITIONAL ANALYSIS

Per Serving: 294 Calories; 22g Fat (3 g saturated fat); 6g Protein; 19g Carbohydrate; 5g Dietary Fiber; 4mg Cholesterol; 103mg Sodium.

"For a non–fish soup eater, this soup tastes great. I'd eat it warm or cold. Does that make me a convert?"

—Stephanie

NOTE

Fennel is also called anise.

Creamy Cauliflower-Zucchini Soup°

Parsley pulls out the subtle flavors of cauliflower and zucchini for a light yet rich soup that's a great starter or a wholesome snack.

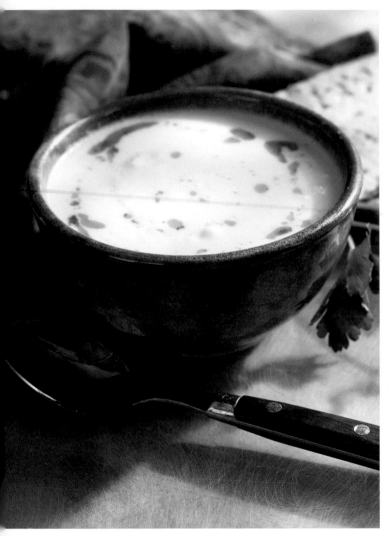

INGREDIENTS

- 1 medium zucchini, peeled and cubed
- 2 cups (200 g) chopped fresh cauliflower tops
- 2 tablespoons (28 ml) olive oil
- 1 teaspoon salt
- 1 tablespoon (14 ml) apple cider vinegar
- 1 cup (235 ml) vegetable broth
- 1 cup (235 ml) water
- 1 large bunch parsley (about ¼ pound, or 115 g), leaves separated from stems

Chop the parsley stems.

In a large saucepan, cook the zucchini and cauliflower in the oil over low heat for about 5 minutes, stirring occasionally. Add the salt, vinegar, broth, and water. Stir for 1 minute then cover and simmer 10 to 15 minutes, until all vegetables are tender.

In a blender or food processor, puree the mixture, adding the parsley leaves in parts. Return the mixture to the pot, cover, and simmer for 5 to 10 minutes. Serve hot or refrigerate overnight and serve chilled.

YIELD: Makes 6 servings.

NUTRITIONAL ANALYSIS

Per Serving: 84 Calories; 5g Fat (1 g saturated fat); 2g Protein; 8g Carbohydrate; 2g Dietary Fiber; trace Cholesterol; 644mg Sodium.

"This tastes so healthy and clean. I feel good eating it."

—Amy

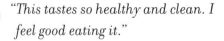

● Loose Stools & Diarrhea ◐ Fiber ◉ Motility and Lubrication ◎ Indigestion ◉ Really Bad Days

On-a-Greens-Kick Soup ○◎

The seeds enable both the flavor and healing properties of this soup. It is also a delicious way to get in a daily serving of greens. Make the recipe on Sunday and serve yourself a portion each day that week.

INGREDIENTS

- 2 tablespoons (28 ml) sesame oil
- 1 teaspoon caraway seeds
- 1 teaspoon sesame seeds
- 1 teaspoon celery seeds
- 1 teaspoon brown mustard seeds
- 2 teaspoons ground ginger
- 4 medium turnips (leaves set aside), chopped
- 1 cup (235 ml) vegetable broth
- 1 cup (235 ml) water
- 1 teaspoon salt
- 1 bunch kale leaves, chopped and stems removed
- 2-4 tablespoons (30-60 g) Homestyle Mustard (page 138) or prepared Dijon mustard

In a deep pot, heat the oil over medium heat and add the caraway seeds, sesame seeds, celery seeds, and brown mustard seeds. Stir-fry the seeds for a minute or two to release scents, but be careful not to burn. Add the ginger and turnips and sauté for 2 to 3 minutes, until the spices coat the turnips. Add the broth, water, and salt. Cover and cook on medium heat for 20 minutes, until the turnips soften. Add the kale, turnip greens, and mustard and continue to cook for another 5 to 10 minutes. Remove from the heat and cool.

Transfer the mixture to a blender in batches and puree. Reheat the pureed soup over low heat just prior to serving; do not boil.

YIELD: Makes 6 servings.

NUTRITIONAL ANALYSIS

Per Serving: 111 Calories; 6g Fat (1 g saturated fat); 3g Protein; 12g Carbohydrate; 3g Dietary Fiber; trace Cholesterol; 782mg Sodium.

"Great taste!" —Robyn

Spinach Balls°°

These delicious and nutritious treats can be prepared ahead and frozen for weeks. Defrost a few to take with you to work. Come 3 o'clock, you'll thank yourself for thinking ahead.

INGREDIENTS

- ¹⁄₃ cup (40 g) ground flaxseeds or flax meal
- ¹⁄₂ cup (120 ml) water
- 1 package (16 ounces, or 455 g) frozen chopped spinach, thawed and drained
- 1 cup feta cheese, crumbled
- 1 cup (155 g) rolled oats
- ¹⁄₄ cup (60 ml) grapeseed oil
- 1 teaspoon cilantro
- 1 teaspoon Homestyle Mustard (page 130) or prepared Dijon mustard

Preheat the oven to 350° F (180°C, gas mark 4).

In a small bowl, combine the flaxseeds or flax meal and water. (The "flax eggs" mixture should form a ball and be slightly sticky.)

In a medium bowl, mix the spinach, cheese, "flax eggs," oats, oil, cilantro, and mustard. Shape the mixture into 1-inch (2.5-cm) balls. Arrange the balls on a large nonstick baking sheet. Bake for 15 to 20 minutes, until lightly browned.

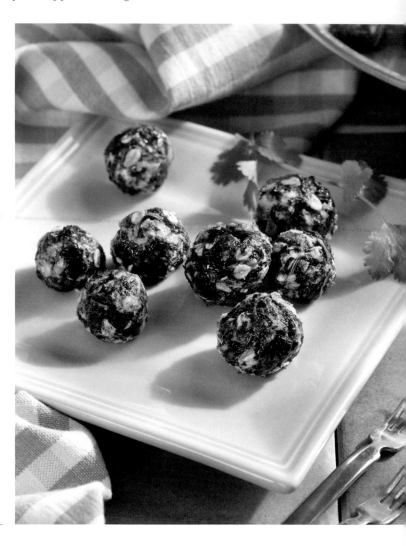

YIELD: Makes 15 servings.

NUTRITIONAL ANALYSIS
Per Serving: 104 Calories; 7g Fat (2 g saturated fat); 4g Protein; 6g Carbohydrate; 2g Dietary Fiber; 9mg Cholesterol; 140mg Sodium.

"Do you think anyone's noticed that I am eating all of these? They're great!"

—Laura

Crab-Pomegranate Rolls©

Pomegranate seeds make these light crab rolls pop with color and flavor. Enjoy them plain or spice it up a bit with the tangy dipping sauce. Pair with Gingerly Twisted Gomasio Sauce (page 133) to improve digestion and enhance motility. My client wanted me to point out that the first time working with rice wrappers can be a bit humbling, but she (as do I) assures you, you're up to the task. It may take a few practice runs to feel comfortable working with the wrappers. Just try it.

INGREDIENTS

- 16 ounces (455 g) fresh lump crabmeat
- Juice of 1 lime
- Seeds from 1/2 pomegranate or 1 cup pomegranate seeds
- 6 rice paper wrappers (6 grams)

In a mixing bowl, combine the crabmeat and lime juice with a fork. Fold in the pomegranate seeds, taking care to not break them open.

Fill a shallow dish with warm water. Submerge one rice wrapper into the water until the water completely covers the wrapper. Let the wrapper soak for 20 seconds. Carefully remove the wrapper with both of your hands. (It will now be very flimsy.) Place the wrapper spread open on a flat surface or cutting board.

Working quickly, scoop 1 to 2 tablespoons of the filling onto each wrapper about a third of the way down. Evenly spread the mixture horizontally across the wrapper, stopping 1/2 inch (1.25 cm) from both edges. Carefully fold the remaining 1/2 inch of the wrapper from each side in toward the center of the wrapper. Then fold the top third of the wrapper down toward the center. (The wrapper should now tightly hold the filling.) Roll the wrapper downward, continuing to do so until the wrapper is completely rolled. Place the roll to the side and begin your next roll. (The wrappers work best when soaked in warm water; as the water begins to cool change to fresh warm water every few wrappers.)

At this point, you can serve the rolls cold. Cut them into thirds and place them on a plate; if storing prior to serving, keep the rolls in a sealed container covered by a damp paper towel or cheese cloth.

If you want to serve the rolls heated, preheat the oven to 350º F (180°C, gas mark 4).

Place the rolls on a nonstick cookie sheet, leaving room between each roll. Bake for 10 to 15 minutes; making sure to rotate the rolls individually every 5 minutes. Remove from the oven and let cool for 5 minutes. Cut into thirds and serve.

"I can't believe how pretty these are that purple. I love the taste too."

—Emma

YIELD: Makes 6 rolls.

NUTRITIONAL ANALYSIS
Per Serving: 84 Calories; 1g Fat (trace saturated fat); 16g Protein; 2g Carbohydrate; trace Dietary Fiber; 67mg Cholesterol; 252mg Sodium.

Sesame-Vegetable Pâté ●◉◎◉ *(constipation)*

This pâté is perfect for entertaining. Dense yet moist, its mellow flavor has universal appeal whether it starts a meal or is part of a buffet spread.

INGREDIENTS

- 2 tablespoons (28 ml) canola oil
- 2 cups (255 g) peeled and diced baby carrots
- 1 cup (85 g) diced fennel
- 2 cups (320 g) chopped sweet onion
- 1/2 cup (15 g) julienned spinach leaves
- 1/2 cup (120 g) canned fire-roasted tomatoes, diced, plus 1/4 cup (60 ml) of its juice
- 1 teaspoon fresh basil
- 1 teaspoon fresh rosemary
- 1 teaspoon fresh thyme
- 1/4 teaspoon mace
- 1/4 teaspoon paprika
- 1 tablespoon (14 ml) balsamic vinegar
- 1/2 cup (120 g) raw sesame tahini
- 2 cups (310 g) rolled oats
- 1 cup (125 g) finely chopped walnuts (optional)

Preheat the oven to 375°F (190°, gas mark 5) degrees. Coat a 9-inch (22.5-cm) square pan with canola oil cooking spray.

In a skillet, heat the oil over low heat and sauté the carrots, fennel, and onion until soft but not brown. Add the spinach, tomatoes, tomato juice, basil, rosemary, thyme, mace, paprika, and vinegar. Lower the heat and cook for 12 minutes. Stir to prevent burning.

Transfer the mixture to a blender and puree. Blend in the tahini.

Transfer the mixture to a bowl and fold in the oats. Transfer the mixture to the prepared baking pan and smooth with a damp knife. Sprinkle the walnuts across the top, if using. Bake for about 30 minutes. Let cool in pan and then cut into squares.

YIELD: Makes 16 (2-inch) squares.

NUTRITIONAL ANALYSIS
Per Serving: 164 Calories; 11g Fat (1 g saturated fat); 5g Protein; 14g Carbohydrate; 3g Dietary Fiber; 0mg Cholesterol; 33mg Sodium.

"I've served this several different ways, hundreds of times, and there has never been any left over."

—Bunny

● Loose Stools & Diarrhea   ◉ Fiber   ◉ Motility and Lubrication   ◎ Indigestion   ◉ Really Bad Days

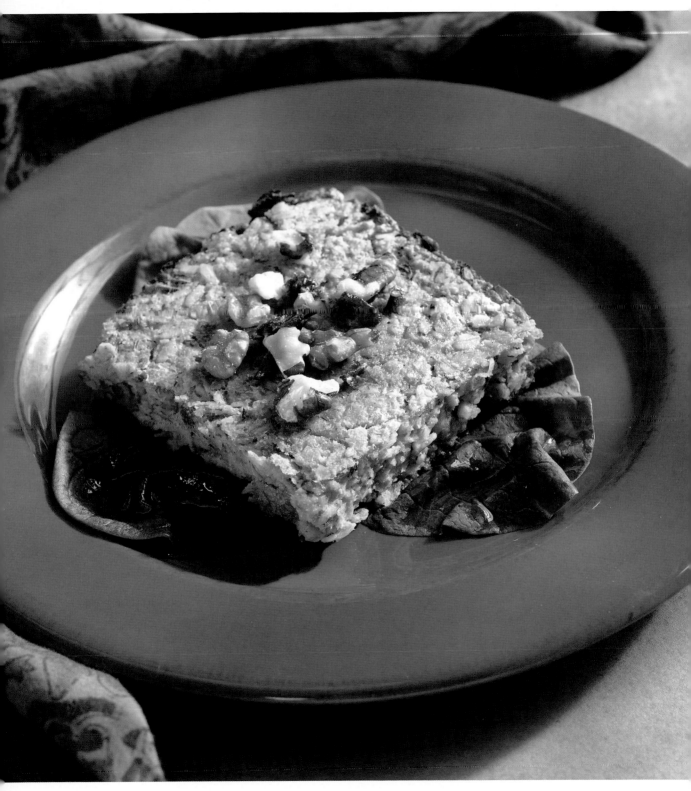

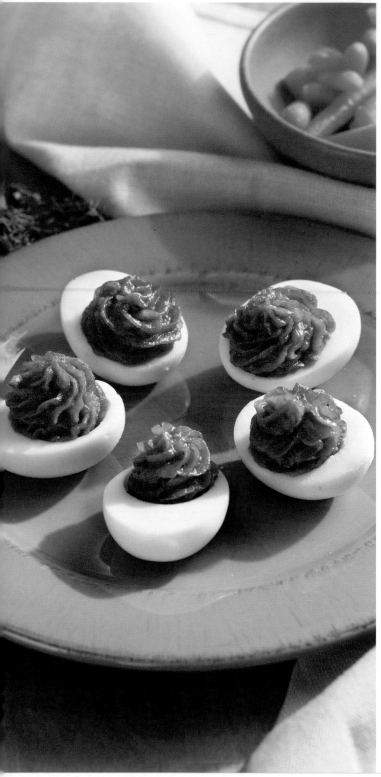

Devilish Eggs

- stuff with sweet potato puree or applesauce
- (diarrhea and constipation)
- try with Prune-Ginger Chutney (page 128)

Ditch the yolks and stuff these eggs with a filling that fits your mood for a quick break-fast, easy snack, or light meal.

INGREDIENTS

- 6 eggs, hard-boiled
- 2 cups (520 g) Tri-Color Salsa (page 126)

Slice the eggs in half and throw away the yolks. Place a tablespoon or so of the salsa where the egg yolk would have been and serve open-faced.

YIELD: Makes 6 servings.

NUTRITIONAL ANALYSIS
Per Serving: 193 Calories; 15g Fat (3 g saturated fat); 8g Protein; 8g Carbohydrate; 2g Dietary Fiber; 212mg Cholesterol; 86mg Sodium.

"I loved these growing up, but I always thought they were bad for me with the mayonnaise. These taste great, and the colors are so fun."

—Sandy

● Loose Stools & Diarrhea   ◔ Fiber   ◉ Motility and Lubrication   Indigestion   Really Bad Days

Savory Pâté ●◎

While the focus of this pâté may be its savory taste, the real story is its quality nutrients. Rich in vitamins such as D and the B complex vitamins, as well as high-quality protein, sunflower seeds tell half the health tale. Their partner in health, sardines, are a noteworthy source of essential fatty acids as well as protein. Consumed with the bones, they are also an excellent source of calcium. Feel good about eating this savory treat.

INGREDIENTS

- ¼ red onion, finely chopped
- 3 teaspoons minced garlic
- 2 tablespoons (6 g) sunflower seeds (see note)
- 1 can (3.75 ounces, or 105 g) wild, **skinless** sardines in olive oil (see note)
- 2 teaspoons lemon juice
- 1 teaspoon oregano
- 7–8 pimento stuffed green olives, drained

Spray a sauté pan with cooking spray and add the onion and garlic. Stir-fry over medium heat for a couple of minutes. Add the sunflower seeds, and cook for 2 to 3 minutes, stirring frequently to avoid burning, until golden brown. Add the sardines and the oil from the can and continue to stir-fry for another 2 to 3 minutes. Remove from heat and let cool.

In a food processor, place the sardine mixture, lemon juice, oregano, and olives and puree into a thick, rich pâté. Transfer to a storage container with a lid; refrigerate for at least an hour. Serve chilled.

YIELD: Makes 6 servings.

NUTRITIONAL ANALYSIS
Per Serving: 76 Calories; 4g Fat (1 g saturated fat); 6g Protein; 4g Carbohydrate; 1g Dietary Fiber; 27mg Cholesterol; 148mg Sodium.

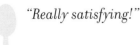

"Really satisfying!"

—Matt

NOTE

I prefer to use fresh sardines where available.

I used Savory Suns sunflowers. Another option is sprouted seeds.

This is delicious on a tortilla or in Zucchini Boat (page 95).

Tang-a-licious Pizza Roll-Ups© omit the cheese

This past December, I sat with a patient to plan food scenarios to help guide her through the holidays. Long struggling with digestive problems, she'd made excellent progress and didn't want the holidays to derail her. As we laid out plans for eating and exercise, one thing seemed to plague her. "I always make the sausage cups. Everyone loves my sausage cups. I have to make them, but they're so bad for you. They will surely make my stomach feel bad. What can I do?" We discussed a few replacements, and presto her classic became a new holiday favorite. "My family and friends didn't even notice the changes, but I felt good about making them healthier, and I could even have a few," she said. Then I had her prepare them for a tasting party; the result? A standing ovation. Now your turn. Enjoy!

INGREDIENTS

- 3 Italian turkey sausage links
- 1 cup (180 g) chopped and drained tomato
- 1/2 cup (80 g) chopped onion
- 2 tablespoons (17 g) minced garlic
- 1/4 cup (10 g) chopped fresh basil
- 1/2 cup (40 g) goat or sheep's milk feta cheese
- 6 rice wrappers

"That's amore!"

—Mike

Remove the sausage meat from the casing as follows. Cut a sliver on either end of the sausage; pinch the center of the sausage link and squeeze the insides out to the left and right of your pinch. Place the contents into a frying pan over a medium heat. Cook the sausage meat completely. (Slice into it to make sure that there is no pink flesh; it should be a grayish colored when cooked.) Remove the sausage from the heat, let sit for 5 minutes, and then drain off any liquid.

Meanwhile, in a mixing bowl, combine the tomato, garlic, onion, and basil. Crumble the cheese into the mixture and fold it in well. Add in sausage and combine well.

Fill a shallow dish with warm water. Submerge one rice wrapper into the water until the water completely covers the wrapper. Let the wrapper soak for 20 seconds. Carefully remove the wrapper with both of your hands. (It will now be very flimsy.) Place wrapper spread open on a flat surface or cutting board.

Working quickly, scoop 1 to 2 tablespoons of the filling onto wrapper about a third of the way down. Evenly spread the mixture horizontally across the wrapper, stopping 1/2 inch (1.25 cm) from both edges. Carefully fold the remaining 1/2 inch of wrapper from each side in toward the center of the wrapper. Then fold the top third of the wrapper down toward the center. (The wrapper should now tightly hold the

● Loose Stools & Diarrhea ◐ Fiber ◉ Motility and Lubrication ◎ Indigestion ◉ Really Bad Days

filling.) Roll the wrapper downward, continuing to do so until the wrapper is completely rolled. Place the roll to the side and begin your next roll. (The wrappers work best when soaked in warm water; as the water begins to cool change to fresh warm water every few wrappers.)

If you want to serve the rolls cold, cut them into thirds and place them on a plate; if storing prior to serving, keep the rolls in a sealed container covered by a damp paper towel or cheese cloth.

If you want to serve the rolls hot, preheat the oven to 350º F (180°C, gas mark 4).

Place the rolls on a nonstick cookie sheet, leaving room between each roll. Bake for 10 to 15 minutes, rotating the rolls individually every 5 minutes. Remove from the oven and let cool for 5 minutes. Cut into thirds and serve.

YIELD: Makes 6 rolls.

NUTRITIONAL ANALYSIS

Per Serving: 244 Calories; 20g Fat (8 g saturated fat); 10g Protein; 4g Carbohydrate; 1g Dietary Fiber; 54mg Cholesterol; 556mg Sodium.

Salmon-Celeriac Salad°

Celeriac, which is also called celery root, may look complicated, but it adds mild, refreshing flavor and a desirable crunch to this salmon salad.

INGREDIENTS

- 1 tablespoon (14 ml) grapeseed oil
- 1 shallot, peeled and minced
- 1 small celeriac, peeled and chopped into bite-size pieces
- 1 teaspoon lemon juice
- 2 teaspoons Homestyle Mustard (page 138) or Dijon mustard
- 1½ teaspoons small capers
- 1 can (6.5 ounce, or 180 g) wild Alaskan salmon, drained

In a saucepan, heat the oil over medium heat. Add the shallot and begin to sauté. After 1 minute, add the celeriac and continue to sauté, until the celeriac softens. Remove from the heat and let cool.

In a small bowl, combine the lemon juice, mustard, and capers. Blend in the salmon, shallot, and celeriac.

YIELD: Makes 4 servings.

NUTRITIONAL ANALYSIS

Per Serving: 120 Calories; 7g Fat (1 g saturated fat); 11g Protein; 4g Carbohydrate; 1g Dietary Fiber; 27mg Cholesterol; 355mg Sodium.

"This is my kind of food—light, healthy, and protein-rich. I'll have it all the time."

—Geoffrey

Hot Vegetable Pie°◎

Warm and filling, this recipe makes an excellent breakfast or dinner on a cold day. For digestive success, it combines two techniques: cooking the vegetables and adding caraway seeds, which reduce the gas-making potential of some healthful foods such as cauliflower, onion, and garlic.

INGREDIENTS

- 1 pie crust (8- or 9-inch, or 20- or 22.5-cm) of your choice (try the Quinoa Crust on page 156)
- ½ cauliflower head (or 2 cups frozen, or 265 g)
- 3 cups (90 g) greens, stems removed (such as collards, spinach, or chard)
- ¼ pound (115 g) fresh mushrooms
- 1 tablespoon (14 ml) canola oil or grapeseed oil, divided
- 1 sweet onion, diced
- 1 clove garlic, minced
- 2 cups (475 ml) milk replacement (curried nut milk recipe or store bought rice, almond, oat 'milk' etc.)
- ⅓ cup (50 g) oats
- ¾ cup (85 g) crumbled goat cheese or sheep's milk cheese (strong flavor)
- 3 teaspoons caraway seeds

Preheat the oven to 425°F (220°C, gas mark 7).

Prepare the pie crust and press it into a pie pan.

Steam the cauliflower and greens until soft. (If using a double pot steamer, place the cauliflower closer to the boiling water, otherwise you may want to steam the cauliflower for a few minutes then add the greens.)

In a frying pan, sauté the mushrooms in ½ tablespoon (7 ml) of the oil over medium heat, until they soften. Pile the cauliflower, greens, and mushrooms into the pie crust and set aside.

Oil the frying pan again with the remaining ½ tablespoon (7 ml) of the oil and sauté the onions and garlic, until they begin to soften.

Meanwhile, in a cup, blend the milk replacement with oats, then combine the mixture in the frying with the onions and garlic. Cook for 1 to 2 minutes, stirring constantly, to thicken. Remove from the heat and stir in the cheese. Pour over the vegetables in the pie crust. Bake, uncovered, for 25 to 30 minutes. Sprinkle the caraway seeds on top and serve.

YIELD: Makes 8 (1-slice) servings.

NUTRITIONAL ANALYSIS
Per Serving: 396 Calories; 20g Fat (4 g saturated fat); 15g Protein; 44g Carbohydrate; 8g Dietary Fiber; 11 mg Cholesterol; 62mg Sodium.

● Loose Stools & Diarrhea ◐ Fiber ◉ Motility and Lubrication ◎ Indigestion ◉ Really Bad Days

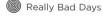

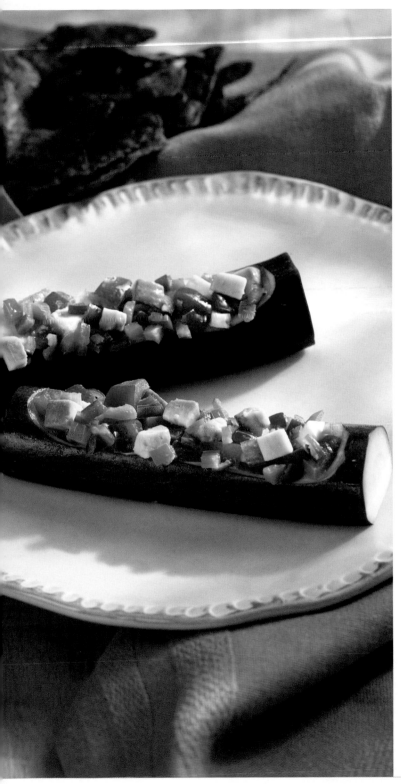

Zucchini Boats°

With their mild flavor, crunchy taste, and ease of digestion, zucchini makes the perfect dipper for your favorite dip or spread. For a taste sensation, try filling them with Savory Pâté (page 91).

INGREDIENTS

- 4 zucchini, washed and ends chopped off

Slice each zucchini in half lengthwise. Lay flat edges on cutting board and cut into thirds (widthwise). Using a vegetable peeler, firmly press the tip of the peeler to scoop out a straight indentation down the center of each zucchini. Serve raw or broiled (lightly sprayed with canola oil).

YIELD: Makes 4 servings.

NUTRITIONAL ANALYSIS

Per Serving: 27 Calories; trace Fat (trace saturated fat); 2g Protein; 6g Carbohydrate; 2g Dietary Fiber; 0mg Cholesterol; 6mg Sodium.

NOTE

Stuff the boats with the dip, salsa, or spread of your choice.

"My kids think these are the neatest. I don't even mind them playing at the table; I'm so happy they're eating vegetables. I let them choose their stuffing. I even put scrambled eggs and salsa in them one morning."

—Marla

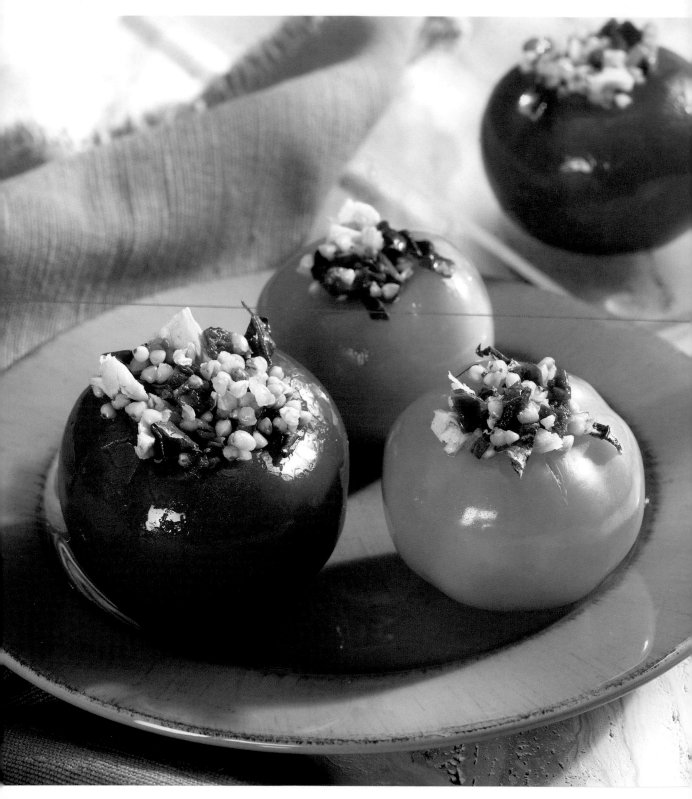

● Loose Stools & Diarrhea ◐ Fiber ◉ Motility and Lubrication ◎ Indigestion ◉ Really Bad Days

Kasha-Stuffed Tomatoes ◎◎

●*omit tomato and serve in bowls* ◎*omit tomato and serve in bowls*

Kasha is the name for roasted buckwheat groats. This gluten-free alternative to wheat (despite sharing a name, they are actually unrelated) delivers fiber and all eight essential amino acids. What's more, according to Chinese medicine, buckwheat helps cleanse and strengthen the gastrointestinal tract.

INGREDIENTS

- 1 cup (165 g) roasted buckwheat groats
- 3 cups (705 ml) water
- 1 teaspoon minced ginger
- 1 teaspoon minced garlic
- 1 zucchini, diced
- 6 sun-dried tomatoes in olive oil, minced
- 3 cups (110 g) diced chard leaves
- 3 cans (6 ounces, 170 g, each) tuna in water, no salt, drained
- ¼ cup (60 ml) balsamic vinegar or apple cider vinegar
- 10 medium tomatoes (not too ripe), preferably different colors

In a large pot bring the groats and water to a boil. Lower the heat and cook, stirring, for 7 to 10 minutes.

In a large saucepan, sauté the ginger, garlic, zucchini, and sun-dried tomatoes. As the zucchini softens, add the chard and continue to sauté. Add the sautéed vegetables to the buckwheat. Cover and simmer, until all of the water is absorbed. Remove from heat and let cool. Blend in the tuna and vinegar to taste.

Wash the tomatoes and remove the tops. Scoop out and discard the seeds. Scoop ¼ of the mixture into each scooped out tomato.

YIELD: Makes 10 servings.

NUTRITIONAL ANALYSIS
Per Serving: 24 7 Calories; 10g Fat (1 g saturated fat); 18g Protein; 26g Carbohydrate; 6g Dietary Fiber; 15mg Cholesterol; 382mg Sodium.

"A meal in a tomato, awesome!"

—Camille

NOTE

If you prefer, you can roast the tomatoes before stuffing them. Cut the tops off and scoop the seeds out first, but don't roast them too long or they will get soggy and collapse.

Over-the-Moon Mini Crab Cakes ◉◉◎

Light and crisp, these little crab cakes make a big impression. Using flaxseeds as a binder adds fiber and taste. But the true difference comes from the sprinkles. They're a true turn-on for any dish, offering visual appeal, texture, taste, and the knowledge that they're good for you too.

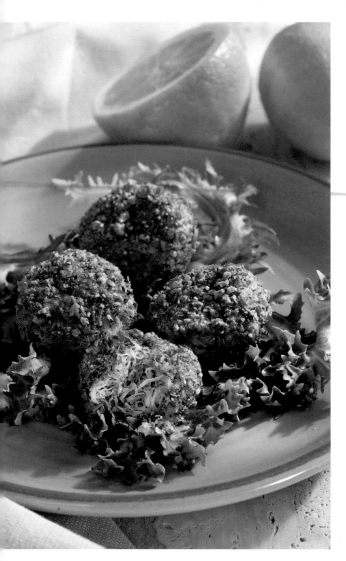

INGREDIENTS

- ¹/₂ cup (80 g) ground flaxseeds
- ¹/₂ cup (120 ml) water
- 1 tablespoon (14 ml) sesame oil
- 1 teaspoon Homestyle Mustard (page 138) or Dijon mustard
- 3 teaspoons minced fresh ginger
- 14 ounces (400 g) lump crab meat
- 2 ounces (55 g) Lydia's Organic Luna Nori Sprinkles or wheat-free bread crumbs

In a food processor, combine the flaxseeds and water into a mayonnaise-like paste.

In a separate bowl, combine the oil, mustard, and ginger.

In a large mixing bowl, place the crab and flax "mayonnaise." Add the oil mixture and combine with your hands.

Place the sprinkles or bread crumbs in a bowl.

Preheat the oven to 350° F (180°C, gas mark 4). Lightly spray a baking sheet with cooking spray.

Pinch out some crabmeat mixture (about the size of an egg yolk) and roll it in the sprinkles or bread crumbs. Place it on the baking sheet. Repeat with the rest of the crabmeat mixture. Bake for 8 to 10 minutes, until golden crisp.

"The flavor is fabulous. I just keep popping them in my mouth."

—Rachel

YIELD: Makes 8 servings.

NUTRITIONAL ANALYSIS
Per Serving: 131 Calories; 6g Fat (1 g saturated fat); 13g Protein; 7g Carbohydrate; 3g Dietary Fiber; 44mg Cholesterol; 224mg Sodium.

● Loose Stools & Diarrhea   ◐ Fiber   ◉ Motility and Lubrication   ◎ Indigestion   ◉ Really Bad Days

Mini Potato Skin Starter ●● *(diarrhea)*

Sometimes it's the package that makes the difference. In this case, the package is not only attractive, but more nutritionally valuable (fiber), than the insides. These skins present an easy, tasty way to serve a dip or spread. Stuff them yourself or let your family or guests stuff their own. The skins are best if prepared the night (or several nights) before serving. Bring your kid into the kitchen and get a little help scooping out the potatoes!

INGREDIENTS

- 1–2 pounds (455 g–1 kg) small redskin potatoes or a variety of potatoes that are similar in size and shape
- 1 teaspoon sea salt

Preheat the oven to 425° F (220°C, gas mark 7). Coat a shallow roasting pan with cooking spray.

Scrub potatoes with a vegetable scrubber. Slice off the top and bottom of each potato so they stand up in the pan. Using a melon-baller or metal teaspoon, scoop out the top end of the potato so a teaspoon or more of filling will set into it. Place the potatoes cut sides down into the roasting pan and roast for 20 minutes, until the potatoes begin to brown and soften but not get mushy. Sprinkle the potatoes with the salt and let cool.

"I love these little guys. I bet my little guys will love them, too."

—Jill

YIELD: Makes 15 servings.

NUTRITIONAL ANALYSIS
Per Serving: 48 Calories; trace Fat (trace saturated fat); 1g Protein; 11g Carbohydrate; 1g Dietary Fiber; 0mg Cholesterol; 146mg Sodium.

NOTE

These are best prepared the night before. Leave the potato skins on the cookie sheet and cover them with foil. Refrigerate. Or you can place them in a freezer-safe container and freeze. To reheat the potato skins, bake them in a 300°F (150°C, gas mark 2) oven, until warm.

Chicken Wrappers ◉◎

Baking chicken en papillote (in parchment) steams while trapping in the flavor. Allow your guests to open their own packets while absorbing the aroma, increasing the pleasure of this light, flavorful appetizer or entrée.

INGREDIENTS

- ⅓ cup (75 ml) sesame oil
- ¼ cup (60 ml) brown rice vinegar
- 2 tablespoons (28 ml) dark agave nectar
- ¼ cup (60 ml) low-sodium soy sauce
- 2 boneless, skinless chicken breasts, 6 ounces (170 g) each, cut into small even pieces, or pre-sliced pieces cut for stir fry
- Parchment paper, cut into 4" (10 cm) squares
- 2 tablespoons (12 g) minced fresh ginger
- 8–10 shitake mushrooms, thinly sliced
- 1 small bunch green onions, rinsed and chopped, discarding tops

Coat a cookie sheet with cooking spray.

In a bowl, combine the oil, vinegar, agave, and soy sauce. Toss the chicken pieces in it; marinate for few minutes, tossing a few times to coat.

Place one square of parchment paper or piece on the diagonal on a flat surface and place chicken piece in lower half. Place a few bits of minced ginger on chicken, lay on a piece of mushroom and a few pieces of green onion. Roll up and twist the ends of the paper to seal the packet and place on a lightly oiled cookie sheet. Continue to wrap rest of bundles, while preheating oven to 425° F (220°C, gas mark 7). Bake for 6 to 8 minutes, checking one packet at 6 minutes. (The chicken should be white but moist and the parchment paper will brown slightly and puff up.) Serve hot and unwrapped.

YIELD: Makes 24 chicken wraps.

NUTRITIONAL ANALYSIS
Per Serving: 55 Calories; 3g Fat (1 g saturated fat); 3g Protein; 3g Carbohydrate; trace Dietary Fiber; 9mg Cholesterol; 108mg Sodium.

"My favorite. The chicken was really moist and had tons of flavor."

—Robin

NOTE

These can be made ahead, partially baked, and reheated before serving. If you're preparing them as a dinner entrée, pound ½ chicken breast for each person and layer as above, using a whole mushroom, wrapping in a 12-inch (30 cm) piece of parchment, and baking for 10 to 12 minutes.

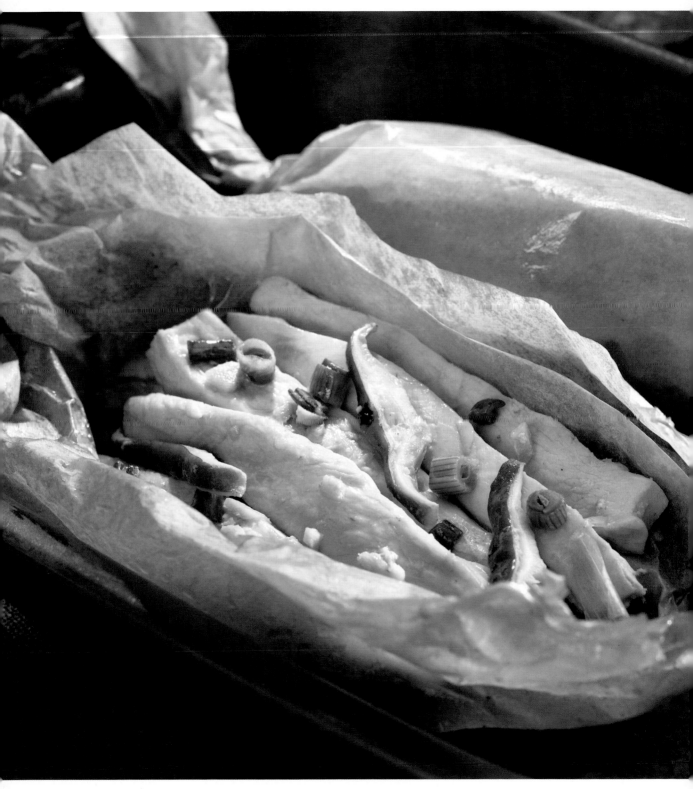

Shrimp-Avocado Cosmopolitan©

Just because something is called salad, doesn't necessarily make it a healthy choice. This holds true for most shrimp, tuna, and egg salads where the protein source often seems an enabler for gobs of mayonnaise. Avocado can replace mayonnaise in almost any uncooked recipe without changing the texture. It significantly improve the quality of a dish and, in my opinion, the taste. Avocadoes are a good source of iron, copper, lecithin, and monounsaturated fat. My mom thought to put this salad in martini glasses.

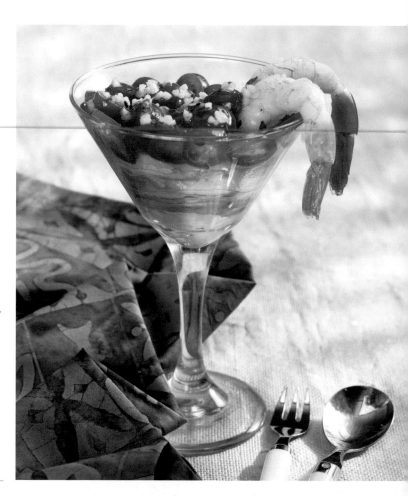

INGREDIENTS

- 2 avocados, peeled and sliced thinly
- $1/2$ pound (225 g) fresh mushrooms thinly sliced (use a mixture, such as shiitake, bella, enoki, etc.)
- 12–18 cooked cocktail shrimp, tails on
- 24 cherry or grape tomatoes, halved
- $1/3$ cup (75 ml) olive oil
- Juice of 1 lemon
- 1 tablespoon (14 ml) white wine vinegar
- 3 teaspoons chopped parsley or chervil
- 1 clove garlic, chopped
- Freshly ground pepper

In a glass bowl or individual martini glasses, layer the avocados, mushrooms, shrimp, and tomatoes.

In a small bowl, whisk together the oil, lemon juice, vinegar, parsley or chervil, garlic, and pepper to taste, to create a vinaigrette. Pour the vinaigrette over the avocado-shrimp mixture. Chill for 1 hour.

YIELD: Makes 6 servings.

NUTRITIONAL ANALYSIS
Per Serving: 259 Calories; 23g Fat (3 g saturated fat); 6g Protein; 11g Carbohydrate; 3g Dietary Fiber; 27mg Cholesterol; 41 mg Sodium.

"Delicious!"

—**Heather**

● Loose Stools & Diarrhea ◐ Fiber ◉ Motility and Lubrication ◎ Indigestion ◉ Really Bad Days

Great Balls of Tempeh °◎

To make tempeh, soybeans are cooked, split, and fermented. This process tends to make tempeh more easily digestible than soybeans. In tempeh, you may find a delicious way to reap the health benefits of soy, which offers all eight essential amino acids and a rich source of omega 3 fatty acid. Toss these balls into a soup, pair them with a vegetable side, or just grab a few for a chewy, crisp, flavorful snack.

INGREDIENTS

- 1 package (8 ounces, or 225 g) tempeh
- ½–¾ cup of your favorite salad dressing (I used Ginger People's Lemon Grass)

Steam the tempeh for 10 minutes. Remove from heat and let cool. Cut the tempeh into bite-size pieces or crumble it. Place it in a shallow pan. Pour the dressing over the tempeh and toss until all pieces are coated with dressing. Marinate for at least 30 minutes, tossing once or twice.

Preheat the broiler. Place the tempeh pieces on a broiler pan and put into the broiler. Broil for 15 minutes, rotating the pieces every 3 to 4 minutes to prevent burning, until each side is crispy and golden brown.

YIELD: Makes 6 servings.

NUTRITIONAL ANALYSIS
Per Serving: 212 Calories; 17g Fat (2 g saturated fat); 7g Protein; 9g Carbohydrate; 0g Dietary Fiber; 0mg Cholesterol; 233mg Sodium.

"You've made a vegetarian very, very happy."

—Mer

NOTE

This recipe can also be made using polenta for people who avoid soy based on dietary preference. Prepare the polenta according to the Polenta-Broccoli-Pesto Pizza recipe (page 47) and cut it into cubes. Marinate the cubes and broil according to the recipe above.

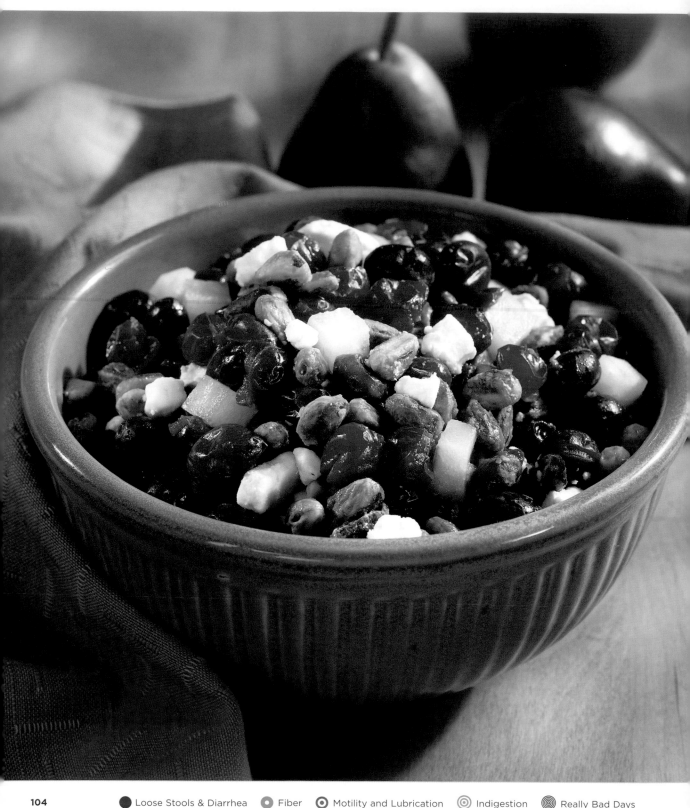

● Loose Stools & Diarrhea ◉ Fiber ◉ Motility and Lubrication ◉ Indigestion ◎ Really Bad Days

Sweet-Tart Baked Cran-Pistachio-Pear Salad

The tartness of cranberries perfectly balance the sweetness of baked pear in this baked salad. Pistachios add color, texture, protein, minerals (potassium, calcium, and iron), and fat. Try this dish as a replacement for traditional cranberry sauce at your next holiday meal.

INGREDIENTS

- 4 pears
- 2 packets (.035 ounce, or 1 g, each) stevia (or alternate sweetener)
- 1 package (16 ounces, or 455 g) cranberries, frozen and thawed or fresh
- 2 cups (250 g) raw, shelled pistachios
- 3 ounces crumbled or cubed goat cheese
- 1 tablespoon (14 ml) plus 1 teaspoon raspberry vinegar

Preheat the oven to 400° F (200°C, gas mark 6).

If you prefer, peel the pears. (Peeling the pears is optional. For more fiber, keep the peel; however, if dealing with a particularly sensitive system remove the peel first.) Place the pears in a 13- by 9-inch (32.5- by 22.5-cm) baking dish. Fill the pan with water up to one-third of the pear. Bake for 20 to 25 minutes, until the pears are tender but not mushy. Let cool.

Meanwhile, add the stevia to a large pot of water on the stove. Bring to a boil and add the cranberries. Reduce to a simmer and stir occasionally, until the cranberries begin to burst open. Remove from the heat, drain, and let cool.

Reduce the oven temperature to 325° F (170°C, gas mark 3).

Cut the pears into small cubes. In a mixing bowl, place the pears and cranberries. Gently fold in the pistachios and cheese. Drizzle the vinegar over the mixture. Transfer the ingredients to the baking dish. Bake for 10 to 15 minutes. Remove from oven, let cool for a minute, and serve warm.

YIELD: Makes 8 servings.

NUTRITIONAL ANALYSIS

Per Serving: 294 Calories; 19g Fat (4 g saturated fat); 9g Protein; 28g Carbohydrate; 8g Dietary Fiber; 9mg Cholesterol; 121 mg Sodium.

"To be honest, I had no idea what to expect. But I love it. It's really flavorful but not heavy."

—Kerri

Mary's Risotto Salad●

This recipe made its way down the block with some replacements to ensure digestive friendliness. The combination of rice and eggplant can be particularly good for people managing chronic diarrhea or loose stools.

INGREDIENTS

- 4 small zucchinis, diced into 1-inch (2.5-cm) cubes
- 2 eggplants, peeled and diced into 1-inch (2.5-cm) cubes
- 1 pound (455 g) cherry tomatoes, halved
- 6 bell peppers, different colors, chopped
- 2 yellow onions, chopped
- 2 garlic cloves, crushed
- 2 tablespoons (28 ml) extra virgin olive oil
- 2 boxes (17.66 ounces, or 494 g, each) Arborio rice for risotto
- 18 ounces (500 ml) low-sodium vegetable broth
- 1/2 recipe Deflate-ing Dressing (page 138)
- 1 package (12 ounces, or 340 g) baby greens
- 10 ounces (280 g) firm goat cheese, cubed (optional)
- 2 teaspoons sea salt

Preheat the oven to 450 º F (230°C, gas mark 8).

Place the zucchini and eggplant in a colander. Sprinkle with the salt and place a weight (such as a ceramic bowl or two wooden spoons) on top. Let stand for 90 minutes. Fluff dry.

In a roasting plan, place the eggplant, zucchini, tomatoes, peppers, onions, garlic, and oil. Roast for 30 to 40 minutes.

Prepare the rice according to the package directions. Heat the broth and add it to risotto.

In a large serving dish, mix the vegetables and risotto with some of the dressing. While the vegetables and risotto are warm, fold in the greens, cheese, if using, and salt. Add more dressing to taste and serve warm.

Makes 12 servings.

NUTRITIONAL ANALYSIS
Per Serving: 517 Calories; 15g Fat (5 g saturated fat); 13g Protein; 83g Carbohydrate; 6g Dietary Fiber; 21 mg Cholesterol; 629mg Sodium.

"The whole neighborhood loves this dish."

—a fan from German village in Columbus, Ohio

● Loose Stools & Diarrhea ◐ Fiber ◉ Motility and Lubrication ◎ Indigestion   Really Bad Days

Red Potato and Green Bean Salad

option: drizzle of olive oil instead of mustard

Mustard helps promote good digestion while providing a nice kick. Try the Homestyle Mustard (page 138) with these mellow vegetables for a pleasant salad.

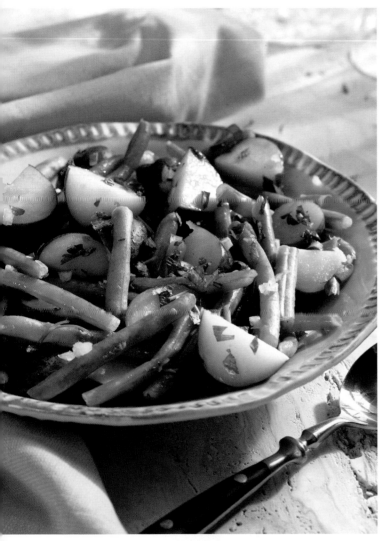

INGREDIENTS

- 8 ounces (225 g) green beans, trimmed and cut
- 3 pounds (1.5 kg) small red-skinned potatoes, scrubbed but not peeled and halved
- 1 shallot, chopped
- 2 tablespoons (28 ml) olive oil (optional)
- 1 cup (240 g) Homestyle Mustard (page 138)
- 2 tablespoons (8 g) chopped fresh parsley
- 2 tablespoons (8 g) chopped fresh mint

Cook beans until they are tender but crisp. (It's ok to do this in the microwave.) Drain the beans and put them in a bowl of ice water to preserve color. Dry on paper towels.

Cook the potatoes in boiling water, uncovered, for 12 minutes. Drain.

In a small bowl, whisk the shallot, oil, and mustard. (You may not need the additional olive oil depending on the consistency of your mustard.) Add the potatoes and toss to coat. Cool completely. Mix in the green beans, parsley, and mint. Cover and refrigerate for at least 10 minutes. Remove from the refrigerator, stir, and let stand for 5 minutes to serve at room temperature.

"Light, not greasy; I like the way this looks and tastes."

—Doug

YIELD: Makes 8 servings.

NUTRITIONAL ANALYSIS

Per Serving: 196 Calories; 5g Fat (1 g saturated fat); 5g Protein; 35g Carbohydrate; 4g Dietary Fiber; 0mg Cholesterol; 388mg Sodium.

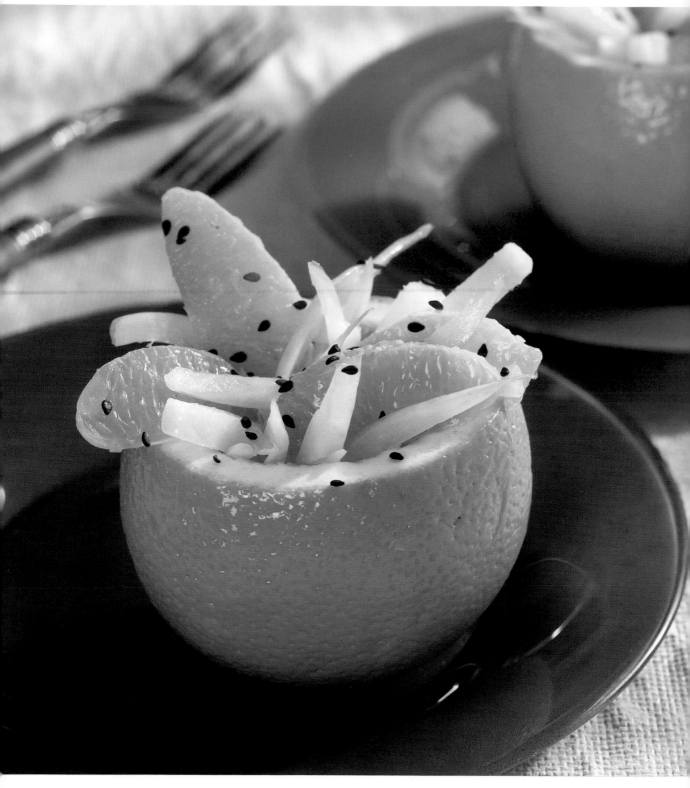

● Loose Stools & Diarrhea ◐ Fiber ◉ Motility and Lubrication ◎ Indigestion ◉ Really Bad Days

Suitable Slaw ◉◎

For most IBS sufferers, cabbage, especially raw, is off limits. And that means coleslaw, a popular favorite, is out, too. Herein lies an alternative that many people find quite suitable. Maybe you'll convert.

INGREDIENTS

- 2 large bulbs fennel
- 1 large or 2 small firm jicama, peeled
- $1/4$ cup (60 ml) grapeseed oil
- 2 oranges, peeled and sliced
- 2 tablespoons (28 ml) olive oil
- 1 teaspoon champagne vinegar
- 2 tablespoons (18 g) black sesame seeds

In a food processor, shred the fennel bulb and the first part of the stem (closest to the bulb, about $1/2$ inch, or 1.25 cm).

In a food processor or by hand, slice the jicama into matchstick slices.

In a large deep-sided frying pan, heat the grapeseed oil over medium heat. Sauté the fennel and jicama, stirring often, until they are firm but softened. (The edges may brown but the vegetables shouldn't stick to the pan.) Once the vegetables begin to soften, add the oranges, continuing to stir gently. After 3 minutes, remove from the heat and set aside to cool.

Meanwhile, in a bowl, whisk the olive oil, vinegar, and seeds together.

Place the fennel mixture in a serving dish (or a mixing bowl if you're serving individually in oranges); toss in vinaigrette, combining well. Serve cold.

YIELD: Makes 6 servings.

NUTRITIONAL ANALYSIS
Per Serving: 245 Calories; 15g Fat (2 g saturated fat); 3g Protein; 26g Carbohydrate; 14g Dietary Fiber; 0mg Cholesterol; 50mg Sodium.

"I don't like fennel, but this was a refreshing summer side. I'm now a fennel convert."

—Stephanie

NOTE

Fennel is also called anise.

For a great presentation, save the whole orange peels or halves and serve the slaw in them.

Sweet 'n Crispy Seaweed Salad°◎● *(constipation)*

For seaweed beginners, wakame offers a sweet flavor that most people will like. Seaweeds are a nutritional powerhouse with many healing properties, including their ability to retain water as they progress through the gastrointestinal tract, thereby adding bulk and lubrication to stools. Wakame is rich in calcium, niacin, and thiamin.

INGREDIENTS

- 2 ounces (55 g) dry wakame
- 1 tablespoon (14 ml) plus 2 teaspoons sesame oil, divided
- 1 tablespoon (14 ml) water
- 1 tablespoon (14 ml) ume vinegar
- ¼ teaspoon crushed ginger
- Zest of ½ lime
- 1 tablespoon (14 ml) dark agave nectar
- 1 cup (95 g) cranberries, cooked
- 1 cup (135 g) pine nuts
- 2 cups (280 g) cubed papaya

In a shallow dish, soak the wakame for 3 to 4 minutes. Drain and cut into strips, removing any thick stems.

In a sauté pan, sauté the wakame in the 1 tablespoon (14 ml) oil and the water over low heat, until the wakame turns crispy. Remove from the heat and set aside to cool.

Meanwhile, in a small bowl, whisk together the vinegar, the 2 teaspoons oil, ginger, lime zest, and agave.

In a saucepan, boil the cranberries until they burst. Drain.

In a larger bowl, toss the wakame, cranberries, pine nuts, and papaya. Drizzle the dressing over the mixture and toss again.

YIELD: Makes 8 servings.

NUTRITIONAL ANALYSIS
Per Serving: 140 Calories; 12g Fat (2 g saturated fat); 5g Protein; 7g Carbohydrate; 1g Dietary Fiber; 0mg Cholesterol; 64mg Sodium.

"I love the seaweed salad. It's so flavorful."

—Yvonne

● Loose Stools & Diarrhea ◐ Fiber ◉ Motility and Lubrication Indigestion 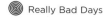 Really Bad Days

Grapefruit-Adzuki Bean Salad ◉◉

Adzuki (or aduki) beans are the most easily digested, thus making them a great place to start for IBS sufferers who've been avoiding beans. Here, the beans meet grapefruit, a fruit known for treating poor digestion, for a light and refreshing taste.

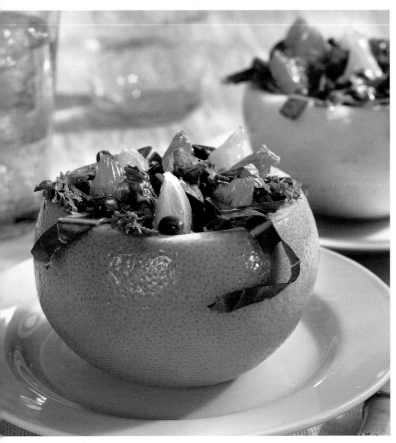

INGREDIENTS

- 6–8 large grapefruits, halved
- 8 ounces (225 g) mixed greens, such as turnip, collard, mustard, and spinach greens
- 2 cups (400 g) dry adzuki beans, cooked and strained, or 2 cups (600 g) canned adzuki beans, rinsed and strained
- 1/4 cup (60 ml) extra virgin olive oil
- 2 teaspoons champagne vinegar

You will be using the grapefruit skin as your 'bowl' so be careful not to poke through it or damage the skin when removing the flesh. It is okay to leave some flesh in the grapefruit. Scoop grapefruit flesh from its peel, remove the seeds, and place in a bowl. (This is easiest if done with a grapefruit knife.)

In a large saucepan with a lid, sauté the greens in the oil for about 4 minutes. Add the beans and continue to sauté until the greens appear wilted. Remove from the heat and add the grapefruit. Drizzle the vinegar on top. Cover and let stand for 10 minutes. Gently toss the mixture and let cool. Stuff each grapefruit skin half and serve.

YIELD: Makes 16 servings.

NUTRITIONAL ANALYSIS
Per Serving: 152 Calories; 4g Fat (1 g saturated fat); 6g Protein; 26g Carbohydrate; 5g Dietary Fiber; 0mg Cholesterol; 5mg Sodium.

"Serving it in a grapefruit, what a great idea!"

—Scott

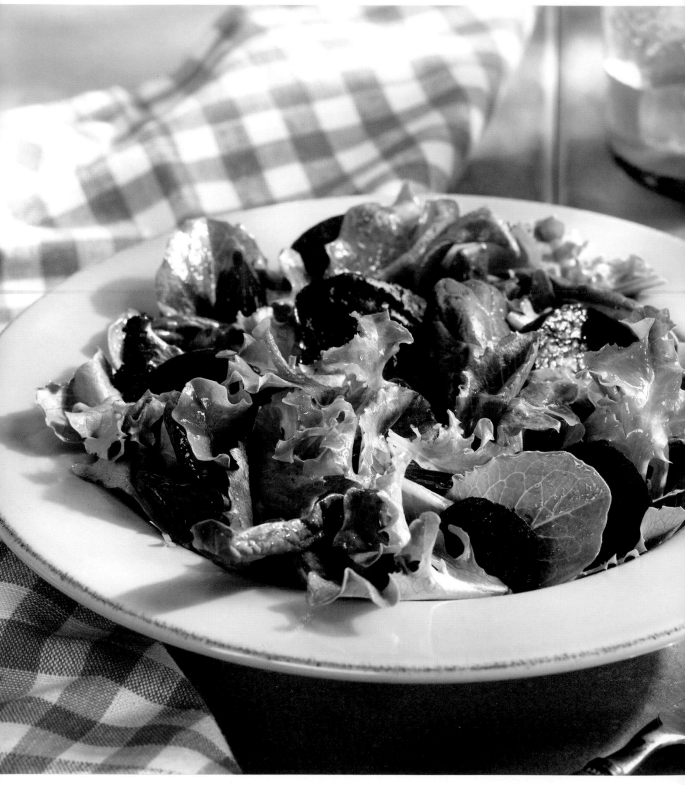

● Loose Stools & Diarrhea ◉ Fiber ◎ Motility and Lubrication ◉ Indigestion ◉ Really Bad Days

Roasted Beet and Blood Orange Salad©

Caraway is especially helpful in the digestion of starches, as well as expelling gas from the digestive tract. Here the seeds offer tanginess to complement the sweetness of the orange and beets.

INGREDIENTS

- 2 medium beets, scrubbed
- 2½ tablespoons (35 ml) olive oil, divided
- 1 blood orange, peeled and cut into bite-size pieces
- 1 cup (30 g) beet greens
- 1 cup (30 g) baby spinach, cut into slivers
- 2 tablespoons (28 ml) raspberry vinegar or balsamic vinegar
- 3 teaspoons caraway seeds
- Salt (optional)

Preheat the oven to 400° F (200°C, gas mark 6).

In a roasting pan, place the beets. Drizzle with 1 tablespoon (14 ml) of the olive oil. Roast for 45 minutes. Cool to room temperature. Peel and cut the beets into bite size pieces. Place beets in a salad bowl. Add the orange, greens, and spinach.

In another bowl, combine the remaining oil with the vinegar, seeds, and salt, if using. Pour over the salad and toss.

YIELD: Makes 6 servings.

NUTRITIONAL ANALYSIS
Per Serving: 78 Calories; 6g Fat (1 g saturated fat); 1g Protein; 6g Carbohydrate; 2g Dietary Fiber; 0mg Cholesterol; 38mg Sodium.

"I love beet salads. This is delicious."

—Jamie

Tuna Krunch Salad©

Kohlrabi and sesame seeds give some crunch to this flavorful tuna salad; they provide digestive (motility) encouragement as well. Kohlrabi also possesses indoles, which may help protect against breast and colon cancers.

INGREDIENTS

- 1 kohlrabi, peeled and cut into bite-size cubes
- 3 cans (6 ounces, or 170 g, each) tuna, in water
- ½ cup (60 ml) canola oil
- 2 tablespoons (28 ml) apple cider vinegar
- 3 teaspoons Homestyle Mustard (page 138) or prepared Dijon mustard
- 3 teaspoons black sesame seeds
- 3 teaspoons Artisan Applesauce (page 132) or prepared unsweetened applesauce

In a large mixing bowl, place the kohlrabi and tuna.

In a small mixing bowl, whisk together the oil, vinegar, mustard, sesame seeds, and applesauce. Drizzle the sauce over the tuna-kohlrabi mixture and gently combine. Only use as much dressing as you need.

YIELD: Makes 6 servings.

NUTRITIONAL ANALYSIS
Per Serving: 192 Calories; 11g Fat (1 g saturated fat); 22g Protein; 1g Carbohydrate; trace Dietary Fiber; 26mg Cholesterol; 320mg Sodium.

NOTES

Water chestnuts can be used if kohlrabi is not available.

Wild canned salmon (such as sockeye), hard-boiled egg whites, or tofu can be used in place of tuna if you don't eat it because of concerns about mercury or dietary preferences.

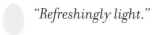

"Refreshingly light."

—Sarah

● Loose Stools & Diarrhea ◔ Fiber ◉ Motility and Lubrication ◎ Indigestion ◉ Really Bad Days

Mung Bean Cakes

roast cumin before using

*Mung beans are one of the most easily digested beans; together with sesame
(tahini) and sunflower seeds, mung beans encourage motility. Cumin
is well known as a digestive aid; when combined with beans it helps to
prevent gas.*

INGREDIENTS

- Grapeseed oil spray
- 1¼ cups (125 g) sprouted mung beans
- ½ cup (65 g) sprouted sunflower seeds
- ½ cup (120 g) raw sesame tahini
- 1 teaspoon ground cumin
- ½ teaspoon salt

*"These little cakes are great
as a midday snack; I took
a few to work."*

—Andy

Preheat the broiler. Spray cookie sheet with oil and set aside.

In a food processor, blend all ingredients. (If you're having difficulty
blending them together, add a teaspoon of water into the mixture.) Spoon
out silver dollar size cakes onto the cookie sheet. Broil for about 2 minutes
on each side, until golden brown. Remove from broiler and let cool.

YIELD: Makes 20 mung bean cakes, or 20 servings

NUTRITIONAL ANALYSIS
Per Serving: 59 Calories; 5g Fat (1 g saturated fat); 2g Protein; 2g Carbohydrate; 1g Dietary
Fiber; 0mg Cholesterol; 61 mg Sodium.

NOTE

*Serve these with mustard or enjoy a few
plain as a snack.*

Sweet Zucchini Pancakes ⊙●◎

The bright color of sweet potatoes hints at the intensity of nutrients this food offers. Rich in vitamin A, the flesh is easily digested and soothing to an irritated digestive system.

INGREDIENTS

- 1 sweet potato, baked and peeled
- 1 zucchini, cut into pieces
- 4 teaspoons teaspoon ground flaxseeds
- ¼ cup (60 ml) water
- ¼ cup (30 g) buckwheat flour
- 1 pinch salt
- Grapeseed oil spray
- 1 tablespoon (14 ml) agave nectar (optional)

In a cup, combine the flaxseeds and water and mix with a fork until it forms a gel.

In a food processor, place all of the ingredients. Blend the ingredients together, leaving the batter slightly lumpy. (Alternately, you could use a mixer. Finely chop the zucchini and mash the sweet potato before combining them with the other ingredients.)

Coat a sauté pan or skillet with grapeseed oil spray and heat over medium-high heat. Using a tablespoon, spoon the batter into the pan or skillet. Flip the pancakes when they turn a darker orange-brown. (Be careful not to burn the pancakes. It is better to flip them frequently.) Let the pancakes cool.

"Four stars. These are the best."

—Robin

Makes 4 servings.

NUTRITIONAL ANALYSIS

Per Serving: 97 Calories; 1g Fat (trace saturated fat); 3g Protein; 20g Carbohydrate; 3g Dietary Fiber; 0mg Cholesterol; 541 mg Sodium.

NOTE

Top with applesauce or avocado spread and enjoy.

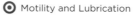 Loose Stools & Diarrhea Fiber Motility and Lubrication 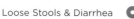 Indigestion 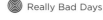 Really Bad Days

Brightly Sautéed Greens ●◐◎◉ *(constipation)*

The ultimate in anti-inflammatory dishes, these greens are a welcome side to any dish or the base of a delicious and bright egg or tofu scramble.

INGREDIENTS

- ¼ cup (60 ml) low-sodium vegetable broth
- 3 tablespoons (18 g) minced fresh ginger
- 1 bag (16 ounces, or 455 g) mixed greens, such as kale, mustard, and collard, stems removed
- 1 teaspoon turmeric
- 1 tablespoon (14 ml) toasted sesame oil

In a saucepan heat the broth and ginger over medium heat. After 1 to 2 minutes, add half of the greens and turmeric and stir until the greens are wilted. Add the remaining half of the greens and continue to stir until all of the greens are wilted. At the last minute, stir in the oil. Remove from the heat and serve.

YIELD: Makes 6 servings.

NUTRITIONAL ANALYSIS
Per Serving: 44 Calories; 3g Fat (trace saturated fat); 2g Protein; 4g Carbohydrate; 3g Dietary Fiber; 0mg Cholesterol; 22mg Sodium

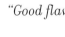

"Good flavor."

—Kathy

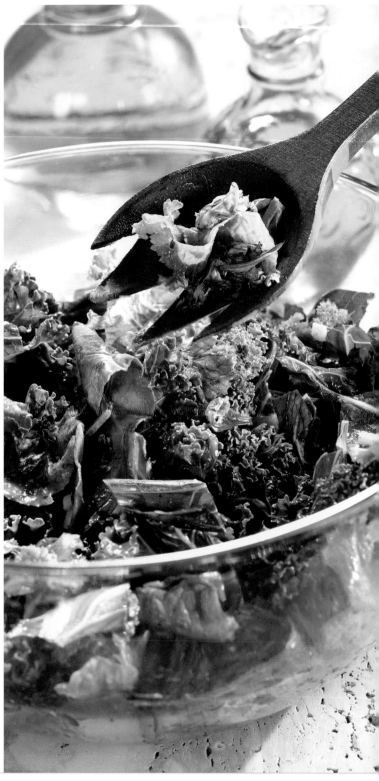

Deeply Greens au Gratin ⊙◉● (constipation)

With the compatible, inviting tastes of coconut milk and Nori Sprinkles, you may not even know you're eating collard greens. This is a perfect side to a piece of fish or paired with another side such as Tang-a-licious Pizza Roll-Ups (page 92) or Mung Bean Cakes (page 115).

INGREDIENTS

- 1 bunch collard greens, washed and stems removed
- ½ cup (80 g) frozen spinach, thawed
- 1 cup (235 ml) light coconut milk
- 2 cloves garlic, peeled and mashed
- 2 ounces (55 g) Lydia's Nori Sprinkles (see note)
- Grapeseed oil spray

Preheat the oven to 400°F (200°C, gas mark 6). Spray a 14 inch (35 cm) oval baking dish with grapeseed oil.

Steam the greens in a steamer for about 6 minutes, until the greens turn bright and wilted.

Meanwhile, in a small saucepot over medium-high heat, bring the coconut milk and garlic to a boil. Reduce the heat and let simmer, stirring to avoid the development of a film. (The coconut milk will thicken or reduce slightly.) Turn the heat off and strain out the garlic.

Place the greens in the bottom of the prepared dish. Pour the coconut milk on top of greens. Spread the sprinkles evenly over the greens-milk combination. Bake for 15 to 20 minutes, until the sprinkles turn golden brown. Remove from oven and let cool 10 for 15 minutes before serving.

YIELD: Makes 6 servings.

NUTRITIONAL ANALYSIS
Per Serving: 133 Calories; 10g Fat (8 g saturated fat); 3g Protein; 10g Carbohydrate; 2g Dietary Fiber; 0mg Cholesterol; 89mg Sodium.

"I had it plain, with some fish, and then with some brown rice. I liked it each time."

—Giovanna

NOTE

These provide delicious flavor and are gluten-free. See "Resources" on page 180 for purchasing information. They can be replaced with crumbled rice crackers or other wheat-free bread crumbs.

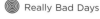

Kristin's Mashed "I Can't Believe It's Not Potato" Cauliflower ○◎

The title says it all. Try it on the kids (maybe skip the garlic and parsley and add some Parmesan), and you'll likely find a new household favorite.

INGREDIENTS

- 1 head cauliflower, tops only, cut into big pieces
- 1 teaspoon salt
- 1 tablespoon (14 ml) garlic oil or olive oil with 2 cloves of garlic
- 1/4 cup (15 g) chopped fresh parsley leaves (optional)

In a deep saucepan, place the cauliflower and salt. Fill the pan halfway with water. Bring to a boil and boil for 10 minutes. Cover the pan, reduce the heat to medium-high, and cook for 20 more minutes. (The cauliflower is done when it's very soft. Poke it with a fork to test before turning off the heat.) Strain the cauliflower very well.

Transfer the cauliflower back into pot and mash it. (If you see water building up at the bottom, put the mashed cauliflower back in the strainer and mash down a few times lightly to remove excess water, then return the cauliflower to the pot.) Add the garlic oil and stir. Sprinkle with the parsley, if using.

YIELD: Makes 8 servings.

NUTRITIONAL ANALYSIS

Per Serving: 35 Calories; 2g Fat (trace saturated fat); 2g Protein; 4g Carbohydrate; 2g Dietary Fiber; 0mg Cholesterol; 289mg Sodium.

Buck-the-Wheat Tortillas ●◎◎ *(diarrhea)*

Buckwheat flour makes these tortillas fairly full-bodied in both taste and texture. A gluten-free alternative, buckwheat delivers fiber and all eight essential amino acids. What's more, according to Chinese medicine, buckwheat helps cleanse and strengthen the gastrointestinal tract.

INGREDIENTS

- 1 cup (110 g) buckwheat flour
- 1/4 cup (60 ml) expeller-pressed canola oil
- 3 teaspoons cinnamon
- 1/2 cup (120 ml) water

Place all ingredients in a food processor and process to form a ball of dough. Divide the dough into eight equal balls. Roll each ball out on wax paper or a floured surface to make a tortilla.

Coat a skillet with cooking spray and heat it over low heat. Place one tortilla on the skillet at a time. Heat for 3 minutes, until the tortilla turns a lighter, sand color. Flip and heat for about another 3 minutes, until light brown on both sides.

YIELD: Makes 10 tortillas.

NUTRITIONAL ANALYSIS

Per Serving: 90 Calories; 6g Fat (trace saturated fat); 2g Protein; 9g Carbohydrate; 2g Dietary Fiber; 0mg Cholesterol; 2mg Sodium.

"These are so easy to make. I love them, and they're gluten-free."

—Maggie

Lentil-Amaranth Pancakes°◉

Lentils are easily digested especially when combined with cumin and pureed. These pancakes use gluten-free amaranth flour, which achieves a more peppery flavor, and also contains an abundance of nutrients, including fiber and lysine, which is an essential amino acid not found in most cereal grains.

INGREDIENTS

- 2 cups (400 g) cooked pink lentils
- 1 cup (110 g) amaranth flour
- 1/3 cup (75 ml) almond oil
- 2 teaspoons cumin
- 1 cup (235 ml) almond milk

In a food processor, combine all ingredients to form a well-mixed dough.

Coat a skillet with grapeseed oil spray and heat over medium-low. Using two teaspoons, place a small amount of batter into the skillet. When the edges begin to brown, flip the pancake over and press it flat with the back of a spatula.

YIELD: Makes 40 mini-pancakes.

NUTRITIONAL ANALYSIS
Per Serving: 57 Calories; 3g Fat (trace saturated fat); 2g Protein; 6g Carbohydrate; 2g Dietary Fiber; 0mg Cholesterol; 2mg Sodium.

"Zesty? Zippy? I'm not sure of the right word, but these have great flavor."

—Rich

● Loose Stools & Diarrhea   ◐ Fiber   ◉ Motility and Lubrication   ◎ Indigestion   ◉ Really Bad Days

"They'll All Root for This" Vegetable Medley●◎

Similar to the veggie chips, it seems people can't get enough of these veggies. Root vegetables are easy to digest and become incredibly sweet when baked. These make an excellent side to an egg scramble or pair nicely with a side like Deeply Greens au Gratin (page 118) for a vegetarian meal.

INGREDIENTS

- 1 teaspoon vanilla extract
- 3 teaspoons cinnamon
- 2 teaspoons ground ginger
- ¼ cup (60 ml) canola oil
- 1 rutabaga, washed, peeled, and cubed
- 2 parsnips, washed, peeled, and cubed
- 4 yellow beets, washed, peeled, and cubed
- 4 red beets, washed, peeled, and cubed
- 1 butternut squash, washed, peeled, and cubed
- 1 turnip, washed, peeled, and cubed
- 2 sweet potatoes, washed, peeled, and cubed (see note)

Preheat the oven to 400º F (200°C, gas mark 6).

In a bowl, whisk together the vanilla, cinnamon, ginger, and oil.

In a shallow, oven- and broiler-safe roasting plan, place the rutabaga, parsnips, yellow beets, red beets, squash, turnip, and potatoes. Pour in dressing and toss, being sure to evenly coat all the vegetables. Bake for 50 to 60 minutes, stirring every 15 minutes with a wooden spoon, until the vegetables soften. Remove from the oven and turn on the broiler. Place the pan in the broiler for approximately 15 minutes, or to desired crispness, stirring the vegetables every few minutes in the broiler to prevent burning.

YIELD: Makes 10 servings.

NUTRITIONAL ANALYSIS

Per Serving: 227 Calories; 6g Fat (trace saturated fat); 4g Protein; 43g Carbohydrate; 9g Dietary Fiber; 0mg Cholesterol; 77mg Sodium.

"What do you do to get these to taste so good? My root vegetables never taste like this."

—EJK

NOTE

You don't have to use these exact vegetables. Choose approximately 3 pounds of root vegetables (weight prior to peeling and cutting). It's best if the vegetables are cubed to about the same size.

Veggie Chips *add broccoli and cauliflower* *add 1 teaspoon dried ginger powder*

 (diarrhea) omit okra and stick with root vegetables

Every time I make these I think I've made enough. And yet every time they're gone within minutes of my serving them. This year's Super Bowl party was no exception. Who knew people would go so crazy for veggies?!

INGREDIENTS

- 1 cup (235 ml) water
- 10 baby carrots, sliced (see note)
- 4 regular or 16 mini zucchini, sliced
- 20 okras, sliced
- 1 bunch Easter egg radishes, sliced
- 2 bunches golden beets, sliced
- Grapeseed oil spray
- 1 teaspoon salt

In a two pot steamer, place the water. Place the beets and carrots in the steamer tray immediately covering the steamer pot. Place the okra, radishes, and zucchini in the steamer tray above the one with the other vegetables. Cover and bring the water to a boil over high heat.

Preheat the broiler. Lightly coat the broiler pan with grapeseed oil spray.

Allow the vegetables to steam for about 6 minutes, until all vegetables soften. Transfer the steamed vegetables to the broiler pan. Lightly coat the vegetables with grapeseed oil spray. Broil for about 10 minutes, flipping the vegetables every few minutes to encourage equal broiling, until the are crispy and golden brown. Sprinkle with salt and serve.

YIELD: Makes 6 servings.

NUTRITIONAL ANALYSIS

Per Serving: 64 Calories; trace Fat (trace saturated fat); 3g Protein; 14g Carbohydrate; 5g Dietary Fiber; 0mg Cholesterol; 413mg Sodium.

"These are Marty's favorite. He can't stop eating them!"

—Barb

NOTE

You can use any vegetables available; the goal is variety in color and shape. The trick here is to slice all your vegetables at about the same thickness. These are an excellent supporting cast for any principle, or they stand alone as a delicious snack.

● Loose Stools & Diarrhea ○ Fiber ◉ Motility and Lubrication ◎ Indigestion 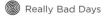 Really Bad Days

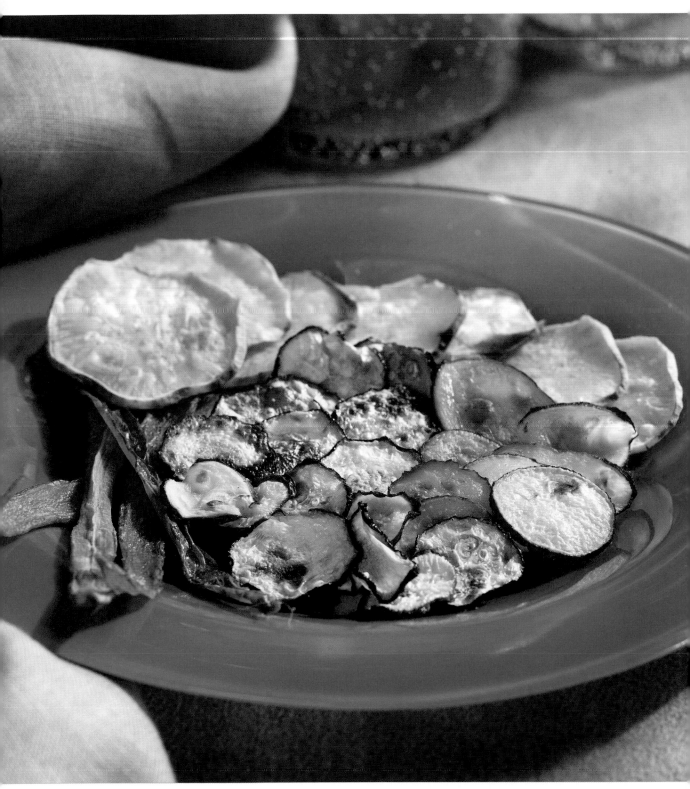

Oat Crackers ○◉●◎◉ *(constipation and diarrhea)*

At Thanksgiving, my sister-in-law introduced me to Nairn's oat crackers. They're a great tasting, high-quality product and the perfect option to comfortably increase the fiber intake. One problem, though, in Los Angeles, I could find them only at The Beverly Hills Cheese shop. I found the idea of sending my IBS clients there a touch too ironic. So while I still recommend finding Nairn's (the good news is they're increasingly more available), I developed this recipe as an option. Keep in mind they are meant to be dense and mellow in flavor; they're perfect for a flavorful dip or spread.

INGREDIENTS

- 2¼ teaspoons active yeast (1 packet)
- 1⅓ cups (310 ml) warm water
- 2 cups (220 g) oat flour
- 1 cup (155 g) steel cut oats
- 1 cup (95 g) oat bran
- 2 teaspoons agave nectar
- 2 tablespoons (28 ml) olive oil
- 4 teaspoons extra virgin olive oil

In a small cup, add yeast packet to the water and let it stand for about 5 minutes, until the yeast dissolves.

In a food processor with a dough blade, place the flour, oats, and oat bran. Blend in the yeast-water mixture and agave. Knead the dough for about 10 minutes, until it becomes elastic. (It may still be a bit sticky.)

Coat a bowl with the oil. Transfer the dough to the bowl and roll the dough in the oil until covered. Cover the bowl with plastic wrap and leave in a mildly warm (70° to 80°F) location for 90 minutes. (The dough will rise slightly, but not significantly.)

Preheat the oven to 425°F (220°F, gas mark 7). Coat a cookie sheet with cooking spray.

Roll the dough out onto a plastic or other nonstick surface. (You shouldn't need to add additional oil.) Cut the dough into squares or triangles. Arrange the crackers on the prepared cookie sheet. Brush crackers with oil. Bake for 20 to 30 minutes, until the crackers are dry and crisp. (The cooking time depends on the thickness and size of the crackers.)

"I really like these, and they do the trick (for me)."

—Anonymous

YIELD: Makes about two dozen crackers.

NUTRITIONAL ANALYSIS

Per Serving: 105 Calories; 4g Fat (1 g saturated fat); 4g Protein; 16g Carbohydrate; 3g Dietary Fiber; 0mg Cholesterol; 1 mg Sodium.

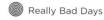

Sesame-Crusted Sweet Potato and Okra Fries ⊚◎

Okra, an excellent source of mucilage (a type of soluble fiber), helps soothe and heal irritation in the gastrointestinal tract. Enjoy these as a tasty alternative to traditional fries and let the healing begin!

INGREDIENTS

- 1 bag (16 ounces, or 455 g) frozen sweet potato spears, unthawed
- 1 bag (16 ounces, or 455 g) frozen chopped okra, unthawed
- 1/2–1 cup (120–235 ml) sesame-ginger salad dressing, such as Ginger People

In a bowl place the potatoes and okra. Add the dressing and toss. Marinate in the refrigerator for at least an hour.

Preheat the broiler. Place the sweet potato and okra on the broiler pan. Broil until they are crispy and golden, flipping frequently to promote equal browning and avoid burning.

YIELD: Makes 8 servings.

NUTRITIONAL ANALYSIS

Per Serving: 207 Calories; 14g Fat (2 g saturated fat); 3g Protein; 19g Carbohydrate; 3g Dietary Fiber; 0mg Cholesterol; 311 mg Sodium.

"This is really tasty. It totally satisfies those French fry cravings."

—Robyn

CHAPTER 4

The Extras:
Dips, Spreads, Sauces, and Beverages

These Extras described above, these recipes add flavor and texture to the Principles and Supporting Cast. They are also important recipes to consider making because store-bought options at a minimum don't often offer the healing ingredients included here within these recipes or in the worst case, contain ingredients that can trigger IBS symptoms.

Tri-Color Salsa°

Lightly sautéing the tomatoes and peppers makes this salsa likely to digest more easily than a raw one. It mixes well with egg whites, such as the Devilish Eggs (page 90) or stuffs nicely into Mini Potato Skin Starter (page 99) or Zucchini Boats (page 95). Tri-Color Salsa's also a key building block in the Build-Your-Own Fish Tacos (page 58). And the addition of avocado makes it like salsa and guacamole all in one.

INGREDIENTS

- 2 cups (360 g) diced mixed color grape tomatoes
- 2 cups (300 g) diced mixed color mini peppers
- 2 tablespoons (28 ml) olive oil
- $\frac{1}{16}$ teaspoon salt
- Black pepper
- 2 ripe avocados, peeled and cut into small cubes

In a mixing bowl, combine the tomatoes, mini peppers (if using), oil, salt, and black pepper to taste.

In a skillet over medium heat, sauté them about 3 minutes, stirring constantly, until the peppers and tomatoes soften slightly. Remove from the heat and let cool for a few minutes. Transfer to a serving dish or a mixing bowl and gently fold in the avocados with wooden spoon.

YIELD: Makes 6 (about $\frac{1}{2}$-cup) servings.

NUTRITIONAL ANALYSIS
Per Serving: 174 Calories; 15g Fat (2 g saturated fat); 2g Protein; 11g Carbohydrate; 3g Dietary Fiber; 0mg Cholesterol; 35mg Sodium.

NOTE

A great alternative to the tomatoes and peppers is zucchini, yellow squash, and apple.

Pineapple Chutney ◎

● *small amounts*

Pineapples contain enzymes, as well as acids known to aid digestion. This chutney uses them as their base for a sweet and powerful spread. Chutney is the perfect companion to bean cakes and turkey slices, or you can even eat it over some greens.

INGREDIENTS

- 1 pineapple, cubed (approximately 2 cups, or 310 g)
- 1/2 bunch fresh cilantro
- 3 teaspoons fresh ginger
- 2 tablespoons (14 ml) fresh lime juice
- 1/4 cup (60 ml) almond milk

In a food processor, blend the juice, almond milk, cilantro, and ginger. Add the pineapple and pulse until the ingredients are well-combined. (It should be chunky.) Strain the mixture over cheese cloth or a fine strainer and serve. Store it in a jar with a tight-fitting lid.

YIELD: Makes about 8 (about 1/4-cup) servings.

NUTRITIONAL ANALYSIS
Per Serving: 47 Calories; 1g Fat (trace saturated fat); 1g Protein; 9g Carbohydrate; 1g Dietary Fiber; 0mg Cholesterol; 1mg Sodium.

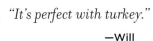

"It's perfect with turkey."

—Will

Omega-3 Pesto ◎◉ *(constipation)*

The name says it all. Hemp seeds, rich in omega 3 fatty acids, also contain GLA (gamma-linolenic acid), a non-essential, but quite useful, omega 6 fatty acid. (Better known sources of it include evening primrose and borage oils.) Hemp seeds also contain an excellent range of essential amino acids. With all this good news, why not give hemp a try? You can buy it at health food stores.

INGREDIENTS

- 6-10 fresh basil leaves, washed
- 1/2 cup (60 g) walnuts
- 2 tablespoons (28 ml) hempseed oil
- 2 tablespoons (30 g) hemp seeds
- 2 pinches salt

In a food processor, chop the basil, adding a little oil to facilitate chopping, if desired. Add the walnuts, hempseed oil, hemp seeds, and salt and process.

YIELD: Makes 16 (about 1-tablespoon) servings.

NUTRITIONAL ANALYSIS
Per Serving: 50 Calories; 5g Fat (trace saturated fat); 2g Protein; 1g Carbohydrate; trace Dietary Fiber; 0mg Cholesterol; 17mg Sodium.

"This is awesome!"

—David

NOTE

The finished pesto is ideally somewhat chunky, but you can play with the ingredient quantities or puree it longer to make a creamier consistency.

Prune-Ginger Chutney ⦿⦾ *(constipation)*

Prunes have a reputation as a natural laxative, to which they live up. Enjoy this spicy, yet sweet chutney and let it work for you.

INGREDIENTS

- 1½ tablespoons (21 ml) canola oil
- 5 shallots, coarsely chopped
- 1 cup (235 g) diced fresh prunes
- 2 tablespoons (28 ml) agave nectar
- 2 tablespoons (28 ml) apple cider vinegar
- 2 teaspoons minced fresh ginger
- ½ teaspoon salt

In a large, heavy saucepan, cook the oil and shallots, stirring occasionally, over medium heat, until the shallots soften. Stir in the prunes, agave, vinegar, ginger, and salt and simmer about 10 minutes, until the prunes soften. Remove from heat and let cool.

YIELD: Makes about 12 (about 2-tablespoon) servings.

NUTRITIONAL ANALYSIS

Per Serving: 62 Calories; 2g Fat (trace saturated fat); trace Protein; 12g Carbohydrate; 1g Dietary Fiber; 0mg Cholesterol; 90mg Sodium.

"This goes great on the lentil pancakes. It's just the right spice."

—Maggie

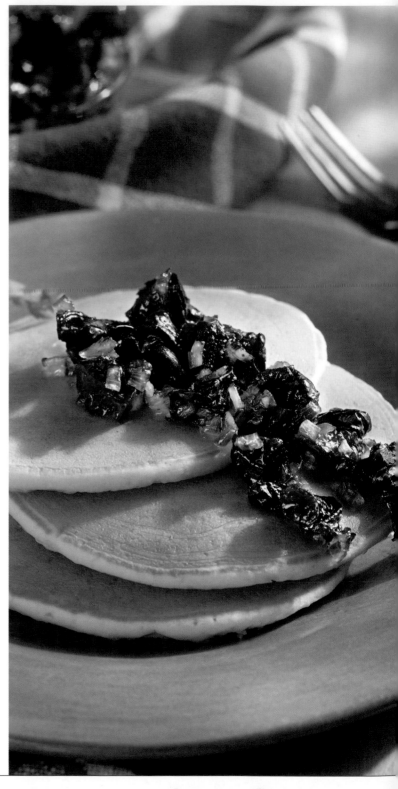

● Loose Stools & Diarrhea ◐ Fiber ◉ Motility and Lubrication ◎ Indigestion ◉ Really Bad Days

Timeless Tapenade

Olives, a fruit, provide a flavor that is at once sweet and sour. Green olives tend to be more acidic so you may want to try black for a milder, yet appreciable flavor, or mix several colors. (I use a variety from an olive bar at the grocery store as opposed to canned or jarred olives.)

Olives are rich in the monounsaturated fatty acid, oleic, making them an acceptable (and delicious) source of fat, in appropriate quantities. Some cultures recommend olives as a healing food for chronic diarrhea.

INGREDIENTS

- 1 cup (135 g) drained and diced pitted olives
- 1 cup (240 g) canned diced roasted tomatoes
- 1/4 cup (14 g) sun-dried tomatoes
- 1/4 cup (60 ml) olive oil (only if the sun-dried tomatoes are not in oil)
- 2 tablespoons (17 g) minced garlic
- Fresh mint or parsley

In a food processor, lightly combine all of the ingredients in a food processor. Garnish with the mint or parsley and serve in a dipping bowl.

Makes 48 (about 1-tablespoon) servings.

NUTRITIONAL ANALYSIS
Per Serving: 15 Calories; 1g Fat (trace saturated fat); trace Protein; 1g Carbohydrate; trace Dietary Fiber; 0mg Cholesterol; 30mg Sodium.

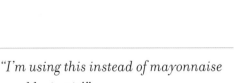

"I'm using this instead of mayonnaise and loving it!"

—Kerry

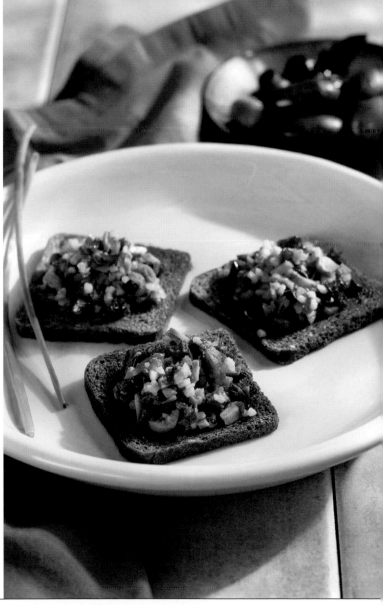

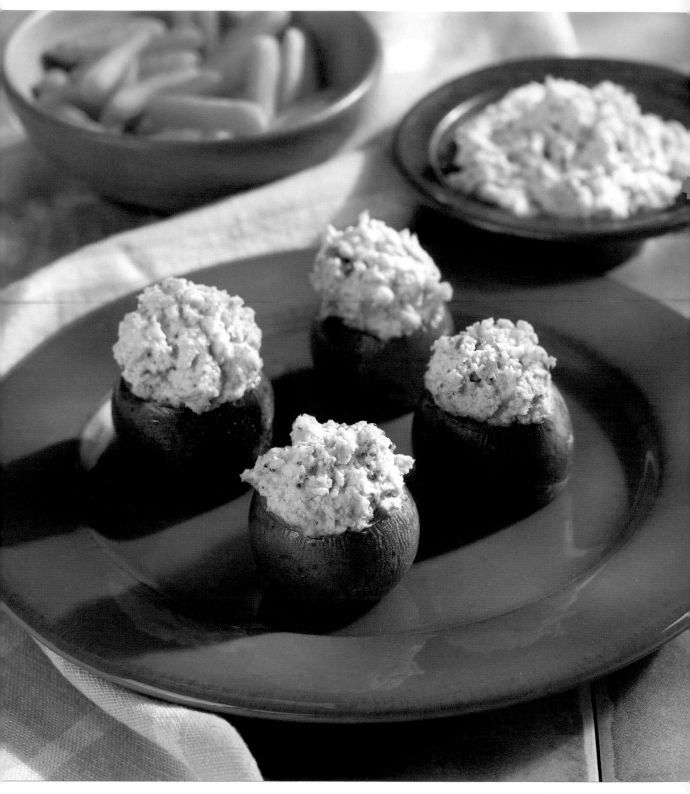

● Loose Stools & Diarrhea   ◐ Fiber   ◉ Motility and Lubrication   ◎ Indigestion   ◉◉ Really Bad Days

Spread the Health°◎

Mentioned earlier, pine nuts provide protein and are mildly laxative. Orange peel is, well, awesome for digestion, and it helps to relieve indigestion and constipation. Here their tangy and nutty flavors perfectly complement broccoli and tofu for a delicately flavored spread. Broccoli and tofu offer calcium, cancer protective nutrients, and fiber (broccoli). Sometimes eschewed by IBS sufferers (sulfur content can promote gas formation), lightly steamed broccoli retains its plentiful chlorophyll, which helps to diminish the unwanted effects of sulfur. So when it comes to broccoli, keep it bright green for health and no gas!

INGREDIENTS

- 1½ cups (135 g) broccoli florets, fresh or frozen, steamed
- ½ cup (70 g) pine nuts, toasted
- 6 ounces (170 g) extra firm tofu (optional)
- Peel of ½ orange
- 1 tablespoon (14 ml) olive oil
- ¼ teaspoon sea salt

Place the broccoli in the top part of a steamer basket and fill the bottom with water. Steam for about 3 minutes, until it turns bright green. Remove it from the heat and allow to cool.

In a food processor, place the broccoli, pine nuts, tofu (if using), orange peel, oil, and salt. Process into a thick spread. (I keep it a bit chunky, but you can further process for a smoother texture.)

"I like the taste. It's a subtle flavor but a good texture"

—Drew

YIELD: Makes 8 (about ¼-cup) servings.

NUTRITIONAL ANALYSIS
Per Serving: 84 Calories; 7g Fat (1 g saturated fat); 4g Protein; 2g Carbohydrate; 1g Dietary Fiber; 0mg Cholesterol; 64mg Sodium.

NOTE

Use this dip with other vegetables, mini-potato skins, or spread on your favorite tortilla for a quick sandwich.

Artisan Applesauce

●   ◉   ◎   ◉

no skins   *(diarrhea and constipation)*   *keep skins*

There are thousands of varieties of cooking and dessert apples. With so many varieties of apples, who could choose just one? Applesauce is a welcome first step back after a really bad day or as a delicious treat any day of the week. So try out different combinations. Be an artist! Your taste buds and GI tract will undoubtedly appreciate your creativity. (See Baked Apples on page 150 for more on the healing power of apples.)

INGREDIENTS

- Baked Apples (page 150)
- 1 teaspoon cinnamon

Prepare the Baked Apples. Let the apples cool then place them and cinnamon in food processor. Process until chunky.

YIELD: Makes 6 (about 1/2-cup) servings.

NUTRITIONAL ANALYSIS
Per Serving: 82 Calories; 1g Fat (trace saturated fat); trace Protein; 21g Carbohydrate; 4g Dietary Fiber; 0mg Cholesterol; trace Sodium.

NOTE

For an alternative, use a combination of pears for "pear-sauce" or combine apples and pears for "apple-pear sauce."

"My kids are going to love this, and so do I."

—Barb

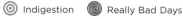

● Loose Stools & Diarrhea   ◉ Fiber   ◉ Motility and Lubrication   ◎ Indigestion   ◎ Really Bad Days

Gingerly Twisted Gomasio Sauce ⊚◎

The idea of combining large amounts of sesame seeds with a touch of salt comes from Japan where this finely ground powder, called gomasio, is frequently used. Here gomasio is the base for a sesame dip that pairs well with grains, crab rolls, and cooked vegetables. From a healing perspective, sesame seeds and oil help lubricate the digestive tract, while ginger contributes valuable anti-inflammatory properties.

INGREDIENTS

- 2 teaspoon black sesame seeds
- Pinch sea salt
- 1 teaspoon ground ginger
- ¼ cup (60 ml) toasted sesame oil

Using a mortar and pestle, grind the sesame seeds and salt into a powder.

Place the ginger and oil in a small bowl and stir to combine. Add the sesame seed mixture and whisk together until the powders fully dissolve.

YIELD: Makes 12 (about 1-teaspoon) servings.

NUTRITIONAL ANALYSIS

Per Serving: 44 Calories; 5g Fat (1 g saturated fat); trace Protein; trace Carbohydrate; trace Dietary Fiber; 0mg Cholesterol; 157mg Sodium.

NOTE

Serve this with Crab-Pomegranate Rolls (page 87) or use it as a dressing for cooked vegetables.

Hemp-Berry Sauce °⊙

Berries, berries, berries. As my pal, the "berry girl," Christine Sardo, M.Ph., R.D., tells it, "The deep color of berries signal their contribution to good health. The powerful synergy of pigments, vitamins, minerals, and fiber in berries may reduce risk for disease."

Hemp is a worthy partner to the berries in taste, appearance, and nutrition. They provide essential fatty and amino acids. Try working with kudzu (or kuzu) as a thickener. Used in Japanese and Chinese cooking, kudzu is soothing to the gastrointestinal tract.

INGREDIENTS

- **3 teaspoons kudzu**
- **1 tablespoon (14 ml) dark agave nectar**
- **¹/₄ cup (60 ml) water**
- **1 package (16 ounces, or 455 g) frozen mixed berries**
- **¹/₄ cup (60 g) hemp seeds**

In a 1¹/₄-quart (1-L) saucepan, prepare the kudzu according to the package instructions. (Dissolve it in cold water first.) Add the agave and water and bring to a boil, stirring. Add the berries. Reduce the heat and simmer for about 10 minutes, until the sauce lightly thickens. Remove from the heat and sprinkle the hemp seeds on top. (Note: Kudzu thickens as it cools.)

YIELD: Makes 8 servings.

NUTRITIONAL ANALYSIS
Per Serving: 66 Calories; 3g Fat (0 g saturated fat); 3g Protein; 7g Carbohydrate; 1g Dietary Fiber; 0mg Cholesterol; 1mg Sodium.

"I know it goes with the toast, but I just want to keep eating it plain. It's sooo good!"

—Maggie

● Loose Stools & Diarrhea   ◉ Fiber   ◉ Motility and Lubrication   ◎ Indigestion   ◉ Really Bad Days
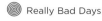

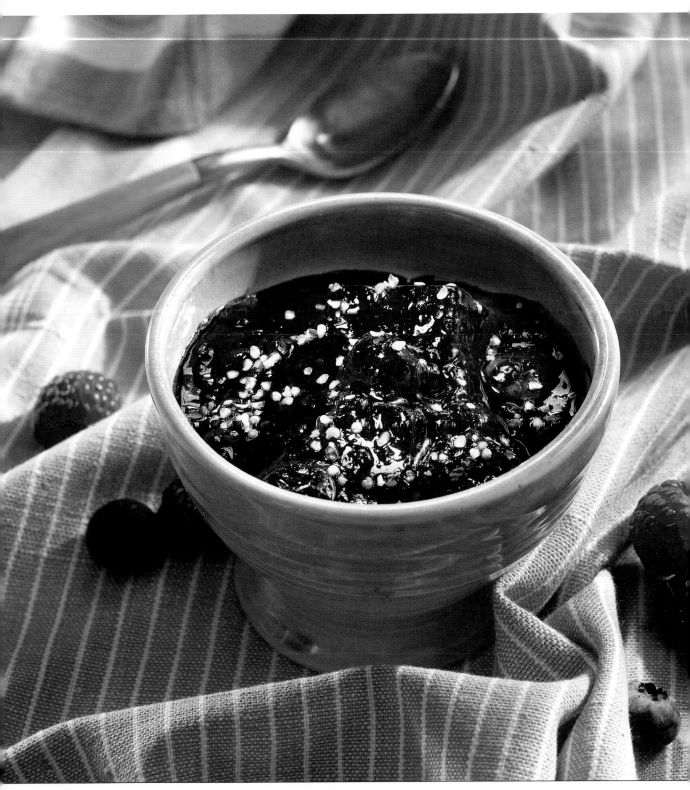

Spinach-Artichoke Dip °

Have you heard? Spinach is good for you. Sure it makes Popeye's muscles strong, but it'll help make your digestive system even stronger by promoting motility and helping reduce inflammation. The problem is that many people don't savor the taste of spinach. But a spinach dip? That's a whole different story. Combined here with artichokes, a light dressing, and some goat cheese, this spinach combo is sure to please.

INGREDIENTS

- 2 tablespoons (28 ml) low-sodium vegetable broth or water
- 1 bag (16 ounces, or 455 g) frozen spinach
- 1 can (13 ounces, or 370 g) artichoke hearts
- ¼ cup (60 ml) favorite dressing (I used Ginger People's Lemongrass.)
- 4 ounces (115 g) goat cheese

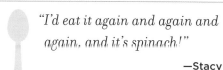

"I'd eat it again and again and again, and it's spinach!"

—Stacy

In a saucepan, heat the vegetable broth or water over medium-high heat. Add the spinach. Cook the spinach until wilted and moist. Strain and let cool.

Preheat the oven to 350°F (180°C, gas mark 4).

In a food processor, place the spinach, artichokes, and dressing. Process and then add the cheese. Pulse to blend in the cheese. Place mixture in a baking dish. Bake for approximately 25 minutes, until the top turns lightly brown. (The exact cooking time will depend on the depth of your baking dish.)

YIELD: Makes 12 (about ¼-cup) servings.

NUTRITIONAL ANALYSIS
Per Serving: 90 Calories; 6g Fat (3 g saturated fat); 5g Protein; 6g Carbohydrate; 3g Dietary Fiber; 10mg Cholesterol; 129mg Sodium.

● Loose Stools & Diarrhea ◉ Fiber ◉ Motility and Lubrication ◎ Indigestion ◉ Really Bad Days

Cashew-Ginger Butter

◉◎

small portions

*Cashews are an excellent source of magnesium—
Mother Nature's masseuse. Magnesium relaxes the
body's muscles, relevant in our case for the muscles
of the digestive system. Here cashews' nutty flavor
receives a sweetly spicy upgrade from ginger.*

INGREDIENTS

- 1 cup (130 g) raw cashews
- ¼ cup (60 ml) canola oil
- 1½ ounces uncrystalized ginger (Trader Joe's), for a sweeter version
- 3 teaspoons ginger powder, for a spicier version

In a food processor, blend all ingredients. (You
may adjust the consistency as desired by the length
of time you process the mixture.)

Makes 24 (about 1-tablespoon) servings.

NUTRITIONAL ANALYSIS

Per Serving: 52 Calories; 5g Fat (1 g saturated fat); 1g Protein;
2g Carbohydrate; trace Dietary Fiber; 0mg Cholesterol; 1 mg
Sodium.

"Yup, this is good."

—Brian

No Más Gas Guacamole◉◎

*Fennel is added to this guacamole for its ability to
reduce flatulence and aid indigestion. Consider
this guacamole an enabler for beans and other gas
makers.*

INGREDIENTS

- 2 tablespoons (28 ml) olive oil or ¼ cup (60 ml) low-sodium vegetable broth
- 2 ripe avocados, peeled and pitted (save the pits)
- ¼ cup (15 g) fresh parsley leaves, stems removed
- 1 fennel bulb, chopped
- Pinch salt
- 3 teaspoons fennel seeds (optional)

In a saucepan, heat the oil or broth over medium-
low heat and sauté the fennel until soft; remove
from heat, and let cool.

In a food processor, place the avocados, parsley,
fennel, and salt. Puree to the desired consistency.
Remove from processor and fold in the fennel
seeds. Serve or store in refrigerator with the
avocado pits to delay ripening.

YIELD: Makes 10 servings.

NUTRITIONAL ANALYSIS

Per Serving: 98 Calories; 9g Fat (1 g saturated fat); 1g Protein;
5g Carbohydrate; 2g Dietary Fiber; 0mg Cholesterol; 31mg
Sodium

"This tastes really fresh."

—Sarah

NOTE

Fennel is also called anise.

Deflate-ing Dressing

to prevent gas and bloating

From the cuisine of North Africa, the dressing called Harissa contains several natural carminatives(foods or spice that help prevents and relieve gas formation in the digestive tract). Use this dressing to help spice up favorites such as Mary's Risotto Salad (page 106) or to lessen the blow of beans or other gas makers.

INGREDIENTS

- 2 tablespoons (13 g) combination of coriander, caraway, and cumin seeds
- ³/₄ cup (175 ml) extra virgin olive oil
- 1¹/₂ rounded teaspoons cayenne
- 3 tablespoons (48 g) (heaping) tomato puree or paste
- 6 tablespoons (90 ml) fresh lime juice

In a dry skillet over medium heat, toast the seeds for 1 to 2 minutes to release their aroma, shaking the pan or stirring with a wooden spoon to keep from burning. Remove from heat and cool; grind the seeds together, using a mortar and pestle or the back of a spoon.

In a mixing bowl, whisk together the seeds, oil, cayenne, tomato puree or paste, and lime juice.

YIELD: Makes 8 (about 2-tablespoon) servings.

NUTRITIONAL ANALYSIS
Per Serving: 190 Calories; 21g Fat (3 g saturated fat); trace Protein; 2g Carbohydrate; 1g Dietary Fiber; 0mg Cholesterol; 32mg Sodium.

Homestyle Mustard

This mustard combines ingredients with positive digestive impact such as turmeric (anti-inflammatory), saffron (digestive aid), apple cider vinegar (potassium, cleansing), olive oil (lubrication), and mustard seeds (combats indigestion).

INGREDIENTS

- 1 tablespoon (14 ml) plus 1 teaspoon dark agave nectar or 2 tablespoons (28 ml) raw honey
- 1¹/₂ cups (355 ml) apple cider vinegar
- Pinch sea salt
- Pinch saffron
- ¹/₄ teaspoon turmeric
- ³/₄ cup (135 g) mustard seeds (you can play with different colors)
- 1–2 tablespoons (14–28 ml) expeller-pressed extra virgin olive oil

In a saucepan, bring the agave or honey, vinegar, salt, saffron, and turmeric to a boil, stirring well. Remove from heat and pour into a food processor or blender. Add the mustard seeds and process. Once the seeds are fully ground into a smooth paste, add the oil to the desired consistency.

YIELD: Makes 32 (about 1-tablespoon) servings.

NUTRITIONAL ANALYSIS
Per Serving: 30 Calories; 2g Fat (trace saturated fat); 1g Protein; 2g Carbohydrate; trace Dietary Fiber; 0mg Cholesterol; 4mg Sodium.

● Loose Stools & Diarrhea ◉ Fiber ◉ Motility and Lubrication ◎ Indigestion ◎ Really Bad Days

A Hummus the Whole Body Will Love ●◉◎

My client suggested that some spices might wake up the mellow tastes of adzuki beans and sesame tahini for a flavorful hummus. And they sure did, with an added health payoff. While adzuki are easily digested (already the most easily digestible beans), in this recipe they become even more so with the addition of cumin. Turmeric and ginger go to work on any inappropriate inflammation. Enjoy this hummus wrapped in a steamed green leaf or as a filler for a Zucchini Boat (page 95).

INGREDIENTS

- 1 can (15 ounces, or 430 g) adzuki beans, rinsed and strained
- 1/3 cup (80 g) raw sesame tahini
- 1 teaspoon turmeric
- 1 teaspoon ground ginger
- 1 teaspoon cumin
- 1 tablespoon (14 ml) lemon juice

In a food processor, place the beans, tahini, turmeric, ginger, cumin, and lemon juice. Pulse to combine but not puree.

Makes 16 (about 1/4-cup) servings.

NUTRITIONAL ANALYSIS
Per Serving: 94 Calories; 3g Fat (trace saturated fat); 2g Protein; 16g Carbohydrate; 1g Dietary Fiber; 0mg Cholesterol; 64mg Sodium.

NOTE

This can stay in the refrigerator for about five days.

ProHydrator ●◉◎◎

Light and refreshing, this beverage combines rich sources of necessary nutrients with digestive-friendliness. Unlike many protein powders, which exacerbated my patients' digestive problems, Jay Robb egg white protein digests easily (thanks to added digestive enzymes) and is a clean (no artificial sweeteners, no preservatives), rich source of highly bioavailable protein. O.N.E. coconut water finally brings to the United States the beverage used throughout the world to manage symptoms of digestive distress by repleting electrolytes. Besides being an excellent source of additional electrolytes, just one serving provides more potassium than a banana. Organic açaí powder delivers phytonutrients to help prevent chronic disease.

INGREDIENTS

- 11 ounces (315 ml) pure coconut water, such as O.N.E.
- 1 scoop (3 g) açaí powder, such as Sambazon
- 1 scoop (28 g) egg white protein powder, such as Jay Robb

In a blender (or in a 16-ounce cup using a hand blender), first add coconut water, then add the powders and blend to desired consistency.

NUTRITIONAL ANALYSIS
Per Serving: 168 Calories; 1g Fat (1 g saturated fat); 26g Protein; 14g Carbohydrate; trace Dietary Fiber; 0mg Cholesterol; 260mg Sodium.

Curried Nut Milk

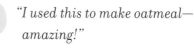

replace the turmeric with ginger powder and fresh mint

This delicious milk or pudding aids in digestion. It's also a tasty milk alternative. Here the recipe calls for soaking and the removal of the skins, heeding the Ayurvedic caution that the skins of almonds may irritate the gut lining.

INGREDIENTS

- 1 cup (145 g) almonds
- 2 tablespoons (14 g) turmeric
- 1 tablespoons (14 ml) agave nectar (optional)
- $^3/_4$ – 1$^1/_2$ cup (175 ml–355 ml) water

> *"I used this to make oatmeal—amazing!"*
> —Andy

Place the almonds in a bowl and cover them with water. Soak the almonds for about 12 hours or overnight. After soaking, drain the almonds, remove the skins, and rub dry.

In a food processor, grind the almonds into a fine meal. Pour into a blender and add the turmeric and agave, if using. Add water ¼ cup (60 ml) at a time while blending. (The amount of water used depends on the desired consistency.)

Makes 4 servings.

NUTRITIONAL ANALYSIS

Per Serving: 236 Calories; 19g Fat (2 g saturated fat); 7g Protein; 13g Carbohydrate; 5g Dietary Fiber; 0mg Cholesterol; 7mg Sodium.

 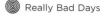

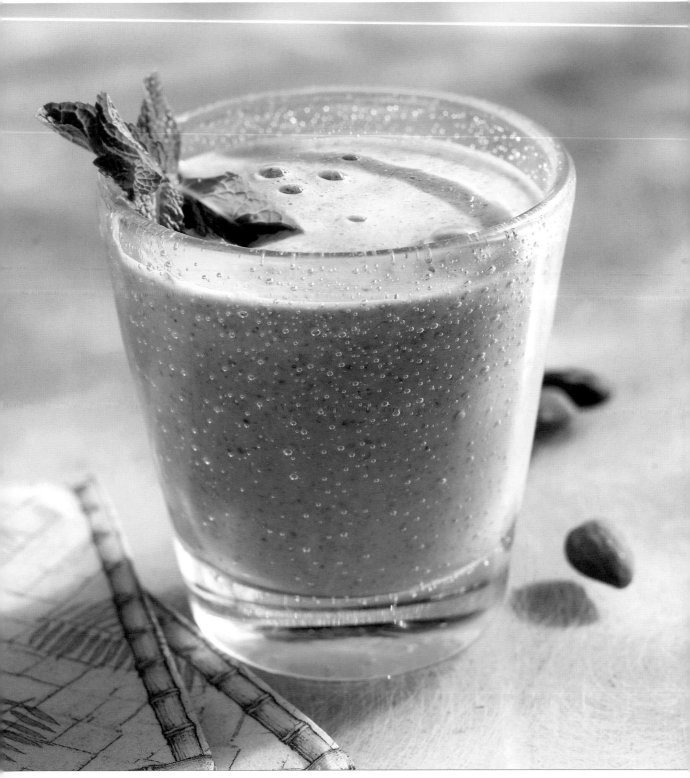

Truly *Naturally* Decaffeinated Tea ○●◎

The health benefits of tea deservedly continue to receive increased attention today. For IBS management, it is appropriate to reduce intake of or avoid caffeine altogether. However, that should not mean missing out on tea and its benefits.

Rather than purchasing decaffeinated teas (whose processing may reduce the healthful constituents of tea), here is a way to significantly reduce the caffeine content of your choice of loose tea or tea bags. It should also be noted that white tea has the least caffeine of true teas, and that there is caffeine in yerba mate.

INGREDIENTS

- 1 tea bag or 1 tablespoon tea leaves
- 8 ounces (235 ml) water

In a cup or heat-safe pitcher, place the tea leaves or tea bags. Bring the water almost to a boil; pour it over the tea bag or leaves. Steep the tea leaves (or bag) by covering the cup with a saucer or plate and let sit for about 30 seconds. Strain the leaves (or tea bag), throw away the water, and re-steep the leaves in fresh boiling or hot water. Your tea is now naturally decaffeinated. Drink it hot or let it cool and then refrigerate it.

YIELD: Makes 1 serving.

NUTRITIONAL ANALYSIS

Per Serving: 5 Calories; 0g Fat (0 g saturated fat); trace Protein; 1g Carbohydrate; trace Dietary Fiber; 0mg Cholesterol; 10mg Sodium.

NOTE

Black, green, oolong, and white teas are actually the leaves of the Camellia sinensis plant. Red tea and herbal teas are not true teas. They are leaves, flowers, and roots of other plants (not Camellia sinensis) and mostly caffeine-free. Some of them—such as peppermint, ginger, and chamomile—may offer benefits to the digestive system, but do not confer the same health benefits as true teas.

See "Resources" on page 180 for In Pursuit of Tea and drweil.com Web sites for more information on tea, its health benefits, and preparation methods.

● Loose Stools & Diarrhea ◐ Fiber ◉ Motility and Lubrication ◎ Indigestion ◉ Really Bad Days
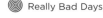

Letting-Go Latte°

Letting go of caffeine and coffee just got a whole lot easier. This hot beverage— sweetly-spiced—should help ease you into a caffeine-free state.

INGREDIENTS

- 6 teaspoons chai tea leaves
- 3 ounces (90 ml) almond milk
- 3 ounces (90 ml) water
- 1 teaspoon dark agave nectar (optional)

In a teapot, place the tea leaves.

In a saucepan, heat the water and milk, until the first sign of a boil, stirring once or twice to avoid a film from developing. Pour the mixture into the teapot. Brew for 3 to 4 minutes. Pour into a mug with a strainer to catch the leaves. Stir in the agave to sweeten, if using.

YIELD: Makes 1 serving.

NUTRITIONAL ANALYSIS

Per Serving: 264 Calories; 14g Fat (1 g saturated fat); 9g Protein; 31g Carbohydrate; 4g Dietary Fiber; 0mg Cholesterol; 43 mg Sodium.

"This is perfect for a bad belly day."

—Marilyn

NOTE

My favorite chai tea is Crimson Chai from www.inpursuitoftea.com, which is caffeine-free. Many chai teas are made from black tea leaves, which do contain caffeine.

Peppermint Sooth-E ●◎

(diarrhea)

Peppermint soothes away indigestion, while rice calms and nourishes. Whether it's a really bad day digestively or emotionally, a glass of Peppermint Sooth-E should relieve any upset.

INGREDIENTS

- 3 cups (705 ml) hot water
- 1 cup (25 g) fresh peppermint leaves
- 2 cups (400 g) cooked brown rice
- 2 teaspoons alcohol-free peppermint oil
- 1 tablespoon (14 ml) agave nectar or maple syrup (optional)

In a saucepan, bring 1 cup (235 ml) of the water to a boil. Remove from the heat and let cool 1 minute.

Place the peppermint leaves in a bowl with a lid. Pour the water over the peppermint leaves. Cover and steep for 8 to 10 minutes.

Meanwhile, in a blender or food processor, blend the rice, remaining 2 cups (475 ml) water, oil, and agave or syrup (if using) until smooth. (The mixture will thicken. Avoid thinning the mixture with additional water.)

Strain the tea, then pour it into the blender. Blend until smooth, removing any lumps, and serve warm or refrigerate.

YIELD: Makes 6 servings.

NUTRITIONAL ANALYSIS

Per Serving: 85 Calories; 1g Fat (trace saturated fat); 2g Protein; 18g Carbohydrate; 1g Dietary Fiber; 0mg Cholesterol; 4mg Sodium.

CAUTION

Mint is not appropriate for people with acid reflux (GERD) as it may exacerbate symptoms.

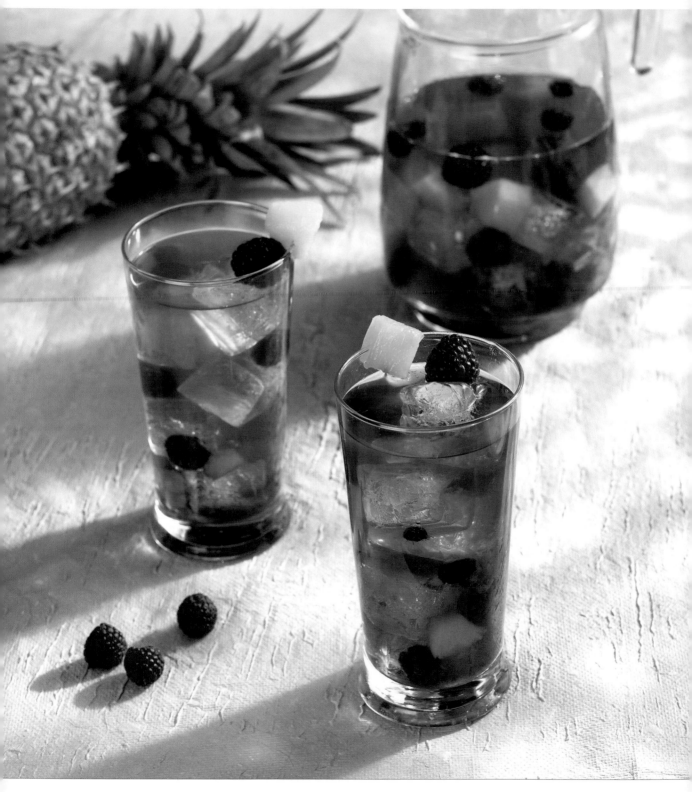

● Loose Stools & Diarrhea ◐ Fiber ◉ Motility and Lubrication ◎ Indigestion ◉ Really Bad Days

Iced Berry Sangri-Tea

(diarrhea and constipation)

Raspberries (and their leaves) as well as their relative, blackberries, help relieve diarrhea. Additionally, all three of the fruits here are good sources of manganese, which helps make those essential fatty acids as well as several enzymes involved in the digestion and metabolism of food.

INGREDIENTS

- 6 cups (1410 ml) water
- 1 cup (25 g) raspberry leaves or 6 tea bags
- 1 tablespoon (14 ml) honey or agave nectar
- 2 cups (500 g) frozen raspberries or blackberries
- 1 cup (245 g) frozen pineapple pieces

Place the raspberry leaves into a tea ball. Place the tea ball or tea bags into a heat-safe glass or metal pitcher.

In a saucepan, bring the water to a boil. Pour it over the raspberry leaves or tea bags in the pitcher. Cover and steep for about 5 minutes. Remove the tea ball or tea bags, blend in the honey or agave and let cool. Place the tea in the refrigerator to chill. Prior to serving, add the raspberries and pineapple to the pitcher, blend with a wooden spoon, and serve from the pitcher.

YIELD: Makes 8 servings.

NUTRITIONAL ANALYSIS

Per Serving: 102 Calories; trace Fat (trace saturated fat); 1g Protein; 26g Carbohydrate; 3g Dietary Fiber; 0mg Cholesterol; 9mg Sodium.

"Light and refreshing, I love the fruit. It's like a mini-meal."

—Monique

Gut Healer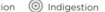

(diarrhea) may want to avoid milk substitute

Many grocery stores and health food stores sell rice protein powders. They are a suitable option for a snack or quick meal that should digest easily. In terms of gut healing, however, there are a few products available at homeopathic pharmacies or through healthcare practitioners (see "Resources" on page 180) that use rice protein powder as a vehicle for nutrients to heal the digestive system. In my practice, I have found these quite useful when food choices are limited, where convenience is needed, and when the patient is likely to benefit from such supplemental nutrients.

INGREDIENTS

- ¹/₄ cup (60 ml) water
- ¹/₄ cup (60 ml) unsweetened milk substitute, such as rice, oat, or almond milk
- 2 scoops (50 g) rice protein powder
- 1 capsule or 1 teaspoon probiotics

In a blender, combine the water, milk substitute, protein powder, and probiotics. (Or mix using a hand mixer.) Drink immediately, but sip slowly.

YIELD: Makes 1 serving.

NUTRITIONAL ANALYSIS

Per Serving: 315 Calories; 10g Fat (1 g saturated fat); 29g Protein; 26g Carbohydrate; 5g Dietary Fiber; 0mg Cholesterol; 30mg Sodium.

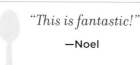

"This is fantastic!"

—Noel

Ginger-AID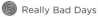

cut back to 3 packets of Emergen-C and do not use sugar-free

It's ginger to the rescue for nausea and general indigestion (not to mention inflammation). For a little bit of fizz (since we're trying to avoid carbonation); orange, lemon, or lime flavor; and a few vitamins, add the Emergen-C. I kept it in a glass bottle in my refrigerator for a few days, and after a workout, or in the mid-afternoon for a non-caffeinated pick-me-up, I shook it up and poured myself a small glass. Quite refreshing.

INGREDIENTS

- 5 tea bags 100% ginger root (I use Triple Leaf Tea)
- 4 cups (950 ml) water
- 1 bottle Ginger Soother (from Ginger People) (optional)
- 5 packets sugar-free Orange Emergen-C or Lemon-Lime

In a saucepan, bring the water to a boil. Pour it into a heat-resistant pitcher, add the tea bags, cover, and steep for at least 10 to 15 minutes. Remove the lid and the tea bags, squeezing the bags as you remove them. Refrigerate the mixture until cold. (You may put it in the freezer to cool more quickly, but stir it with a wooden spoon occasionally to avoid ice developing.) Once cold, add the Ginger Soother, if using, and Emergen-C. Whisk together and serve.

YIELD: Makes 6–8 servings.

NUTRITIONAL ANALYSIS

Per Serving: 0 Calories; 0g Fat (0 g saturated fat); 0g Protein; 0g Carbohydrate; 0g Dietary Fiber; 0mg Cholesterol; 4mg Sodium.

Iced Revelation ◉◎ *in place of coffee for coffee drinkers*

Many IBS sufferers (constipation dominant) use coffee to, well, stimulate the bowels. Without going into all the reasons this may not be a solution for long-term health, I present an alternative. Ready for a revelation? Teecino's ingredients include chicory, a known digestive stimulant. Perhaps Iced Revelation is just what you need to make the switch from coffee.

INGREDIENTS

- 2 tablespoons (20 g) Java Teeccino
- 2 tablespoons (20 g) Hazelnut Teeccino
- 8 cups (1000 ml) water

Combine the two types of Teeccino and brew according to package directions. Let cool. Place in a metal bowl or pitcher in the freezer. After 20 minutes, stir it to break up any ice forming on the top. Remove after an hour. Serve cold.

YIELD: Makes 8 servings.

NUTRITIONAL ANALYSIS
Per Serving: 0 Calories; 0g Fat (0 g saturated fat); 0g Protein; 0g Carbohydrate; 0g Dietary Fiber; 0mg Cholesterol; 7mg Sodium.

NOTE

See "Resources" on page 180 for Teeccino information.

"I'm surprised by how much I liked this because I love coffee."

—Anne-Marie

CHAPTER 5

The Finales:
Desserts

Yes, these are desserts. But they can also steal the show as a snack to brighten up your morning or afternoon. Enjoy.

Divine Berry Crisp°

Synonyms for divine include heavenly, celestial, lovely, and blissful. According to feedback I received, this dish warrants its name. Hemp provides essential fatty acids and amino acids, berries help protect against disease, and ginger lends its anti-inflammatory properties for quite a finale. See Hemp-Berry Sauce (page 134) and Ginger-AID (page 146) recipes for additional health information. Plus, with Divine Berry Crisp, you can make use of those leftover berries in your refrigerator!

INGREDIENTS

- 3 cups (750 g) frozen berries, defrosted and drained
- 1 cup (100 g) finely chopped crystallized ginger
- ⅓ cup (75 ml) sparkling water
- ½ cup (120 ml) maple syrup or agave nectar
- 1 cup (120 g) Where-for-Heart-Thou Granola (page 172) or store-bought granola such as Lydia's Organic or Bear Naked

Preheat the oven to 350°F (180°C, gas mark 4). In a baking pan, combine the berries and ginger. In a bowl, combine the water and maple syrup or agave. Pour over the berry-ginger mixture. Spread the granola over the berries. Bake for 30 to 40 minutes.

YIELD: Makes 10 servings.

NUTRITIONAL ANALYSIS
Per Serving: 203 Calories; 6g Fat (1 g saturated fat); 2g Protein; 37g Carbohydrate; 2g Dietary Fiber; 0mg Cholesterol; 12mg Sodium.

"Oh my!—in a good way."

—Chris

 Loose Stools & Diarrhea Fiber Motility and Lubrication 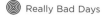 Indigestion 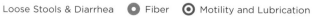 Really Bad Days

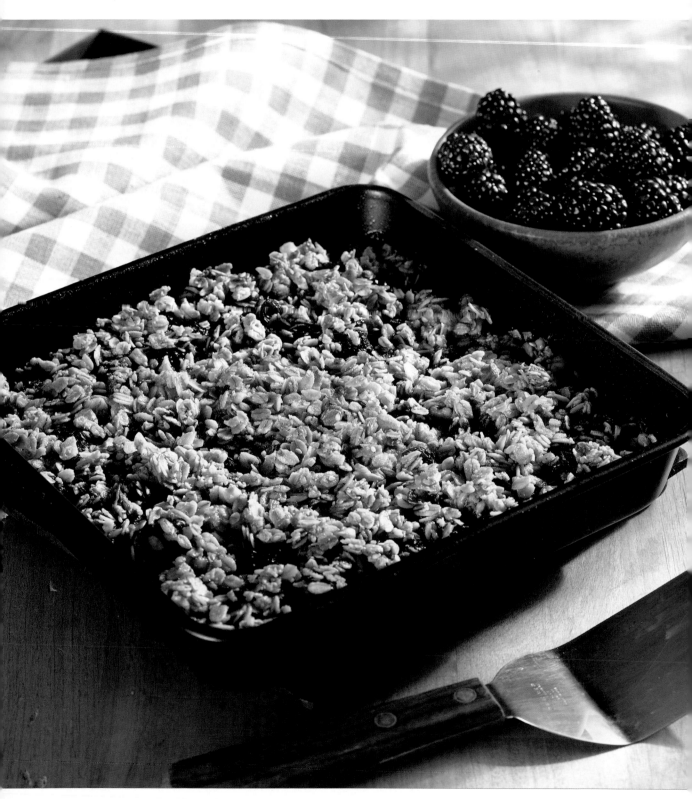

Baked Apples ●● ○◎

(diarrhea and constipation) without skins   *with skins*

Apples are the digestive tract's best friend. They help to create a hospitable environment for good bacteria (prebiotic), they contain acids that help keep bad bacteria homeless, and their pectin also acts as a bulking agent. Here baking increases the sweetness for a warm, easily digestible snack or treat.

INGREDIENTS

- **6 organic apples, washed (see note)**

Preheat the oven to 400°F (200°C, gas mark 6).

Core the apples if you'd like. In a baking pan, arrange the apples so that they are not touching each other or the sides of the pan. Fill pan with water until approximately one-third of the apple is covered. Bake for 30 to 40 minutes, until the skin is golden brown. Remove the pan from the oven, drain the water, and let cool.

YIELD: Makes 6 servings.

NUTRITIONAL ANALYSIS

Per Serving: 81 Calories; trace Fat (trace saturated fat); trace Protein; 21g Carbohydrate; 4g Dietary Fiber; 0mg Cholesterol; 0mg Sodium.

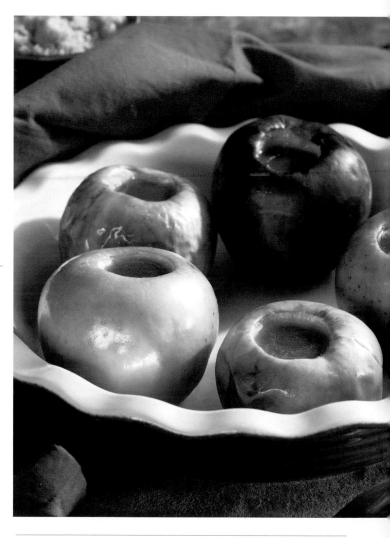

NOTES

It is best if the apples are about the same size. Baked apples will keep for 3 to 5 days in the refrigerator.

For baked pears, follow the same instructions, noting that pears typically require less cooking time.

"I've been eating one of these every day since I met Ashley (over a year ago). I love them. I used to eat a muffin as a treat, but this is my treat now. And I feel good. Amazing!"

—Marilyn

Nobody's Rhubarb Fool ⚫◉◎◉ *(constipation)*

You won't feel foolish for choosing this finale. Rhubarb, which is actually a vegetable, sweetens as it cooks; it also offers laxative properties. Orange peel is, well, awesome for digestion, and it helps to relieve indigestion and constipation. Rice bran beats out oat bran for soluble fiber content nearly two to one; it's a must for IBS sufferers and here it works parfait-ly with rhubarb and orange peel.

INGREDIENTS

- 8 stalks rhubarb, ends removed and cut into $\frac{1}{2}$-inch (1.25-cm) pieces (see note)
- 2 tablespoons (28 ml) dark agave nectar
- Juice and peel from 1 orange (ideally organic)
- $\frac{1}{2}$ cup (60 g) rice bran, divided

In a saucepan over medium-low heat, bring the rhubarb, agave, orange peel, and orange juice to a boil. Reduce the heat to low and simmer for about 6 minutes, partially covered, until the rhubarb softens considerably. Blend in $\frac{1}{4}$ cup (30 g) of the rice bran and stir until it has dissolved into rhubarb mixture. Continue to simmer, partially covered, stirring occasionally, until most of the rhubarb pieces dissolve. (The mixture will thicken considerably with the addition of the rice bran.)

Meanwhile, coat a small skillet with cooking spray. Add the remaining $\frac{1}{4}$ cup (30 g) of rice bran and toast over low heat, until the rice bran turns a bit crispy and darkens in color.

Remove the rhubarb and rice bran from the heat and set aside to cool. In individual bowls or glasses, layer the rhubarb and rice bran to make a parfait.

YIELD: Makes 8 servings.

NUTRITIONAL ANALYSIS

Per Serving: 53 Calories; 2g Fat (trace saturated fat); 1g Protein; 11g Carbohydrate; 2g Dietary Fiber; 0mg Cholesterol; 3mg Sodium.

"I really like this, and I usually don't like healthy desserts!"

—Mer

NOTE

Look for pinkish to red (ideal) stalks.

Banana Pudding

● *(diarrhea) use less ripe bananas*

◉ *use very ripe bananas and rice bran*

Bananas, carob, and sweet rice flour easily digest and help heal the diges-
tive tract. Bananas help to support the good bacteria of the digestive tract.
Their ripeness will affect their impact on the bowel: less ripe tend to bind
up, whereas more ripe are more laxative. Eat this plain, as a pudding, as a
stuffing for your favorite mochi, or as a sauce drizzled over baked apples.

INGREDIENTS

- 3–4 bananas, peeled
- 2 teaspoons carob powder
- 3 teaspoons brown rice sweetener
- ¼ cup (30 g) sweet rice flour
- ½ teaspoon xantham gum
- 1 teaspoon vanilla
- 3 teaspoons rice bran (optional)

In a food processor or blender, combine all ingredients and process or
blend to the desired thickness.

YIELD: Makes 8 servings.

NUTRITIONAL ANALYSIS
Per Serving: 89 Calories; 1g Fat (1 g saturated fat); 1g Protein; 20g Carbohydrate; 2g Dietary
Fiber; trace Cholesterol; 2mg Sodium.

"MMMMmmmmmm, yummy; my daughter likes it
too (she's 18 months)."

—Sally

● Loose Stools & Diarrhea ● Fiber ◉ Motility and Lubrication ◎ Indigestion ◉ Really Bad Days

Digestif-ly Pleasing Poached Pears ●◐◎◉ *(constipation)*

Pears stand out for digestive treatment because they contain water-soluble fiber (even more pectin than apples). There are several different varieties, with Comice typically touted as the sweetest and most flavorful. Bitters are a 'digestif' often taken before meals to enhance digestion.

INGREDIENTS

- 4 firm pears (not too ripe), peeled and halved
- 2 ounces (60 ml) bitters
- 2 tablespoons (28 ml) agave nectar
- 2 tablespoons (28 ml) lime juice
- 1 teaspoon allspice
- 1/2 cup (120 ml) water

In a saucepan big enough to hold the pear halves, combine all ingredients except the pears. Cover and bring mixture to a boil. Reduce the heat and simmer for about 3 minutes. Place the pears in the saucepan, cover, and poach over low heat, flipping them every few minutes, for about 10 minutes, until tender. Turn off the heat and let the pears cool in the covered pan. Refrigerate to chill and serve on a bright colored plate with a sprig of mint.

YIELD: Makes 4 servings.

NUTRITIONAL ANALYSIS
Per Serving: 137 Calories; 1g Fat (trace saturated fat); 1g Protein; 35g Carbohydrate; 4g Dietary Fiber; 0mg Cholesterol; 1 mg Sodium.

"I'd like to serve these to guests because they are so pretty and taste good, but they are healthy too."

—Rose

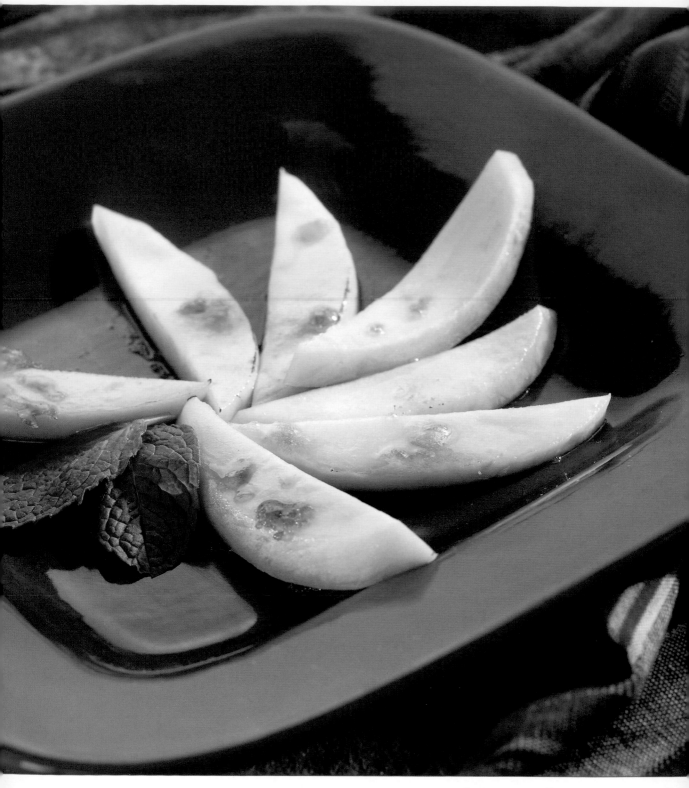

● Loose Stools & Diarrhea   ◔ Fiber   ◉ Motility and Lubrication   ◎ Indigestion   ◉ Really Bad Days

Mango Carmelitas°

Bob, a family friend and fabulous chef, started something good here. Simply sultry, and sweet, this fruit stands alone as a dessert, or you can partner it as a sweet addition to a "Jerk" Turkey Burger (page 65) or Deeply Greens au Gratin (page 118).

INGREDIENTS

- 1 mango, peeled and sliced thinly
- 2 tablespoons (28 ml) balsamic vinegar
- 2 teaspoons grapeseed oil
- 2 tablespoons (20 g) light brown sugar or 1 tablespoon (14 ml) agave nectar

Preheat the broiler.

Place the mango on a broiler rack. In a bowl, whisk together the vinegar and oil. Drizzle mixture over mango slices, then sprinkle with sugar. Broil for about 2 minutes, until golden brown.

YIELD: Makes 4 servings.

NUTRITIONAL ANALYSIS
Per Serving: 92 Calories; 3g Fat (trace saturated fat); trace Protein; 19g Carbohydrate; 2g Dietary Fiber; 0mg Cholesterol; 3mg Sodium.

"This is super sweet, just the way I like it."

—Sam

Gluten-Free Pie Crust ●◉◎◉

Easy to make, this gluten-free (and wheat-free!) pie crust makes a great foundation for pies or bars.

INGREDIENTS

- ¹/₂ cup (55 g) oat flour
- ¹/₂ cup (55 g) sweet rice flour
- ¹/₄ teaspoon salt
- ¹/₄ cup (60 ml) canola oil
- 2–3 tablespoons (28–45 ml) ice water

Preheat the oven to 400°F (200°C, gas mark 6). Lightly flour a 9-inch (22.5-cm) pie pan.

In a medium mixing bowl, combine the oat flour, rice flour, and salt. Fold in the oil, using your fingers to mix. Add the water, 1 tablespoon at a time, using as little as necessary to hold the dough together without it becoming sticky.

Press the dough into the prepared pie pan and flute the edges with your fingers or the back of a fork. Bake for 10 to 15 minutes, until it lightens up but doesn't turn brown, or bake for 5 minutes and then add pie filling and continue to bake following the pie recipe's directions.

YIELD: Makes 1 pie crust.

NUTRITIONAL ANALYSIS
Per Serving: 1074 Calories; 61g Fat (5 g saturated fat); 18g Protein; 115g Carbohydrate; 10g Dietary Fiber; 0mg Cholesterol; 536mg Sodium.

Quinoa Crust ◎◉

Pile on the veggies (as in hot vegetable pie) or your favorite fruit (like Austin's Grandmum's Quince Pie, page 158).

INGREDIENTS

- 1¹/₂ cups cooked quinoa
- 1 teaspoon xantham gum
- ¹/₄ cup (30 g) rice bran
- 2 tablespoons (30 g) macadamia nut butter
- 2 tablespoons (28 ml) dark agave nectar
- 1 teaspoon cinnamon

Preheat the oven to 400°F (200°C, gas mark 6). Lightly coat an 8-inch (20-cm) pie pan with cooking spray.

In a food processor, combine all ingredients. (Do not overprocess; the dough should be well combined but not appear whipped.) Spread the dough into the prepared pie pan. Use the back of a fork to create edges. Bake for 15 to 20 minutes and then add pie filling and continue to bake following the pie recipe's directions (if you will be cooking again with pie filling) or bake for about 30 minutes if you will not be cooking any longer.

YIELD: Makes 2 pie crusts.

NUTRITIONAL ANALYSIS
Per Serving: 1361 Calories; 37g Fat (6 g saturated fat); 43g Protein; 23 3g Carbohydrate; 23g Dietary Fiber; 0mg Cholesterol; 60mg Sodium.

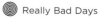

Momentous Fig Bars °◉

These delicious treats are likely to build a little digestive momentum as well thanks to the known natural laxative power of figs.

INGREDIENTS

- 1 cup chopped dried figs
- 1 packet (100 g) frozen acai or 2 cups other frozen berries
- 1 cup (235 ml) milk substitute, such as rice or almond milk
- 2 tablespoons (14 g) sweet rice flour
- ¼ teaspoon salt
- ½ cup (50 g) steel cut oats
- 1 Gluten-Free Pie Crust (page 150) (baked in a square pan; pressed flat; no fluting)

Preheat the oven to 350ºF (180°C, gas mark 4). In a medium saucepan, combine the figs, acai or berries, milk, flour, and salt and simmer until the mixture thickens.

In a skillet or on baking sheet, lightly toast the oats. Pour the fig mixture into the crust and sprinkle the oats on top. Bake for 30 to 40 minutes, until the fig mixture gels together. Let cool and cut into squares.

YIELD: Makes 20 bars.

NUTRITIONAL ANALYSIS
Per Serving: 107 Calories; 5g Fat (trace saturated fat); 2g Protein; 13g Carbohydrate; 2g Dietary Fiber; 0mg Cholesterol; 54mg Sodium.

"These are good for me, too?!"

—Erika

Austin's Grandmum's Quince Pie°◎

Thanks to Camille and Jon for Austin, and thanks to Jennifer for Austin's quince. Who knew how good cooked quince tastes and how good it is for digestive complaints?! Here's a pie from our family to yours.

INGREDIENTS

- 3 ripe quinces; peeled, cored, and sliced
- 3 teaspoons sugar or 1 tablespoon (14 ml) light agave nectar
- 1 orange, thinly sliced
- 1 Gluten-Free Pie Crust (page 156) or ½ Quinoa Crust (page 156)
- ¾ cup (175 ml) lemon juice

Preheat oven to 350°F (180°C, gas mark 4.)

In a square baking dish with a cover (or use foil), place a layer of quince. Next, sprinkle some sugar or agave on top of the quince and cover with a layer of orange slices. Continue to layer. Pour the lemon juice over the layers, cover, and cook for 90 to 120 minutes, until the quince softens. (Test it after 90 minutes with a fork.) Remove it from the heat and let cool. Reserve a few quince and orange slices for garnish.

In a blender or food processor, place the remaining quince and orange slices. Blend or process briefly to create a thick pie filling. Spread mixture into the crust and garnish with the reserved quince and orange slices. Bake for about 10 minutes, until the filling gels and the crust edges turn slightly golden. (The cooking time will depend on the type of pie crust used.) Remove from the heat and let cool. Serve as a pie or cut into squares and enjoy as bars.

> *"He likes quince; that was my mum's idea."*
>
> —Camille

YIELD: Makes 12 slices.

NUTRITIONAL ANALYSIS

Per Serving: 116 Calories; 5g Fat (trace saturated fat); 2g Protein; 17g Carbohydrate; 2g Dietary Fiber; 0mg Cholesterol; 46mg Sodium.

● Loose Stools & Diarrhea ◔ Fiber ◉ Motility and Lubrication ◎ Indigestion ◉ Really Bad Days

Bunny's Baked Fruit Medley°°

Mom makes it best—plain and simple. But here you can try your hand at a family favorite.
Enjoy it plain or sprinkle on some hemp seeds for an even more nutritious crunch.

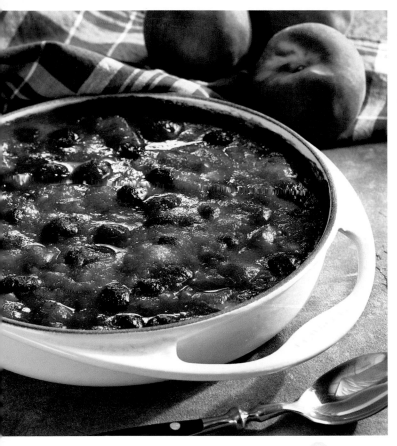

INGREDIENTS

- 1 bag (10 ounces, or 280 g) frozen cherries.
- 1 bag (10 ounces, or 280 g) frozen peaches
- 2 ripe mangoes, peeled and diced
- Assortment of other frozen fruits or fresh fruit, peeled and cut, such as 2 cups berries, 1 cup papaya (or ½ papaya), and 2 cups pineapple
- 1 jar (4 ounces, or 115 g) unsweetened applesauce
- 2 teaspoons almond extract

Preheat the oven to 325°F (170°C, gas mark 3). Lightly spray a 2- to 3-quart (2- to 3-L) ovenproof serving bowl with grapeseed oil spray.

Run frozen the fruits in their bags under cold water, just to separate but not defrost. In a large mixing bowl, combine the fruits and gently stir in the applesauce and almond extract. (Use more or less applesauce based on the amount of fruit.) Pour the mixture into the serving bowl. (At this point, it can be covered and refrigerated overnight.) Bake uncovered for 40 minutes.

YIELD: Makes ½-cup servings. (The number of servings depends on amount of fruit used.)

NUTRITIONAL ANALYSIS
Per Serving: 49 Calories; trace Fat (trace saturated fat); trace Protein; 12g Carbohydrate; 1g Dietary Fiber; 0mg Cholesterol; 2mg Sodium.

NOTE

This keeps well in the refrigerator and reheats easily.

"I loved the baked fruit. It's so warm and filling."

—Sally

Stewed Figs

While not true eye candy, these dried figs impart elaborate flavor for a sweet and tangy mouth candy. Figs not only provide the natural laxative power for which they are well-known, but also work with "the good guys" (good bacteria) to fend off the "bad guys." Enjoy them alone or over goat's milk yogurt.

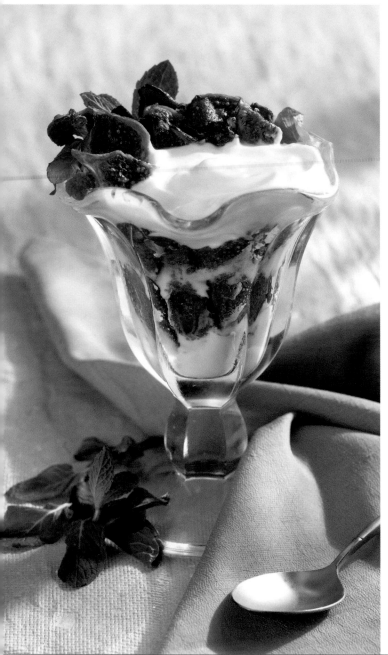

INGREDIENTS

- 1 tablespoon (14 ml) dark agave nectar
- 1 tablespoon (14 ml) balsamic vinegar
- 1¼ cups (295 ml) water
- ¼ cup (6 g) fresh mint leaves
- 15 dried Calimyrna figs
- 15 dried Black Mission figs

In a saucepan, combine the agave, vinegar, and water and bring it to a boil. Add the mint and figs, cover, and simmer for 5 to 10 minutes, until the figs are very soft. Place 6 figs with some of the mint into glass dessert bowls.

YIELD: Makes 5 servings.

NUTRITIONAL ANALYSIS
Per Serving: 305 Calories; 1g Fat (trace saturated fat); 4g Protein; 78g Carbohydrate; 14g Dietary Fiber; 0mg Cholesterol; 16mg Sodium.

> "I wasn't going to, but I'm glad I did. Yum."
>
> —Claudia

Kiwi Kream ©

Kiwis are less well known than papaya and pineapple as a source of useful digestive enzymes that help break down protein. They can even curdle milk. No worries here, though, as this dairy-free ice cream alternative pairs kiwi with lime and macadamia for a refreshing, sweet cream replacement. Some people even recommend eating acid fruits (like lime and kiwi) with proteins (such as nuts) at the same meal.

INGREDIENTS

- 4 ripe kiwis, peeled
- Juice from ½ lime
- Peel from ½ lime (optional)
- 1 tablespoon (14 ml) dark agave nectar
- 3 teaspoons sweet rice flour
- 2 tablespoons (30 g) macadamia nut butter

Follow the instructions to prepare your ice cream maker. (They typically require placing the bowl in the freezer at least 24 hours prior to use.)

In a food processor or blender, combine the kiwis, agave, and lime juice and blend until the kiwis are completely pureed. Thicken by adding sweet rice flour a teaspoon at a time. Place the mixture in an ice cream maker and blend. When ready, scoop Kiwi Kream into small bowls, drizzle with macadamia butter (which tends to be thinner than other nut butters), and garnish with lime peel, if using.

YIELD: Makes 6 servings.

NUTRITIONAL ANALYSIS
Per Serving: 79 Calories; 3g Fat (1 g saturated fat); 2g Protein; 15g Carbohydrate; 2g Dietary Fiber; 0mg Cholesterol; 3mg Sodium. Exchanges: 0 Grain (Starch); 0 Lean Meat; 1/2 Fruit; 1/2 Fat.

"I just need a little taste to satisfy my sweet craving."

—Jenna

NOTE

If you cut the kiwis in half and scoop the flesh out (as opposed to peeling) you can use the kiwi skin halves as your serving dishes. Place them in the freezer while you prepare the Kiwi Kream.

14-Carrot Ice Cream°

Carrots just moved out of the vegetable bin and into the favored world of frozen delights. Coconut adds a nice chewy crunch to this golden treat.

INGREDIENTS

- 3 cups (375 g) sliced carrots
- 1 teaspoon vanilla extract
- 1/2 cup (125 g) smooth almond butter
- 1/4 cup (20 g) shredded coconut
- 1 tablespoon (14 ml) dark agave nectar

Follow the instructions to prepare your ice cream maker. (They typically require placing the bowl in the freezer at least 24 hours prior to use.) It's best to prepare the ice cream mixture the night before as well.

Steam the carrots and let cool.

In a food processor, blend the carrots, vanilla, almond butter, coconut, and agave. Prepare the ice cream according to the instructions of your ice cream maker.

Makes 6 servings.

NUTRITIONAL ANALYSIS

Per Serving: 182 Calories; 14g Fat (2 g saturated fat); 4g Protein; 14g Carbohydrate; 3g Dietary Fiber; 0mg Cholesterol; 24mg Sodium.

Snappy Ginger Cookies°◎

Snap your fingers, and you'll have ginger cookies the whole family will love. Quick to make and more moist than traditional ginger snaps, Snappy Ginger Cookies employ the healing power of ginger to reduce inflammation and settle digestive distress.

INGREDIENTS

- 2 cups (220 g) oat flour
- 1/2 cup (60 g) flax meal
- 2 tablespoons (12 g) crystallized ginger
- 1 teaspoon ground ginger
- 1 teaspoon baking powder (ideally aluminum-free)
- 1 teaspoon baking soda
- 1/2 cup (120 ml) maple syrup
- 1/4 cup (60 ml) blackstrap molasses
- 1/2 cup (125 g) unsweetened applesauce

Preheat the oven to 350°F. Lightly coat a cookie sheet with cooking spray.

In a mixing bowl, blend together the flour, flax meal, ginger, baking powder, and baking soda. Mix in the ginger, syrup, molasses, and applesauce. Use two teaspoons to scoop out and place spoonfuls of batter onto the prepared cookie sheet. Bake for 12 to 15 minutes.

YIELD: Makes 30 cookies.

NUTRITIONAL ANALYSIS

Per Serving: 78 Calories; 2g Fat (trace saturated fat); 2g Protein; 14g Carbohydrate; 2g Dietary Fiber; 0mg Cholesterol; 62mg Sodium.

"I love carrot cake, and now, I love carrot ice cream!"

—Petra

"I can't believe this is a vegetarian option. My kids will be thrilled."

—Geeta

● Loose Stools & Diarrhea ◐ Fiber ◉ Motility and Lubrication ◎ Indigestion ◉ Really Bad Days

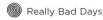

Pistachio-Coco Cream©

As a child, I recall watching my dad shell and eat pistachios and always thought "That's a bit of work!" but they must be worth it. Indeed they are. Pistachio's unique flavor and texture make it a favored nut around the world. Here it combines with coconut milk and lemon for a light flavor but substantive cream. Enjoy this cream on an oat cracker or as a snack all alone. Raw pistachios help alleviate slowed bowel function.

INGREDIENTS

- 1 cup (125 g) shelled pistachios
- 2 teaspoons fresh lemon juice
- 1/3 cup (75 ml) light coconut milk

In a food processor, place the ingredients and process until creamy. Store in the refrigerator.

YIELD: Makes 4 servings.

NUTRITIONAL ANALYSIS
Per Serving: 235 Calories; 21g Fat (6 g saturated fat); 7g Protein; 9g Carbohydrate; 4g Dietary Fiber; 0mg Cholesterol; 5mg Sodium.

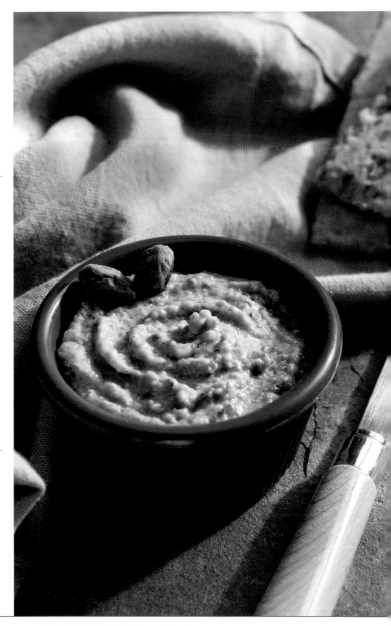

"Yeah. I can have an ice cream now—sort of!"

—Monique

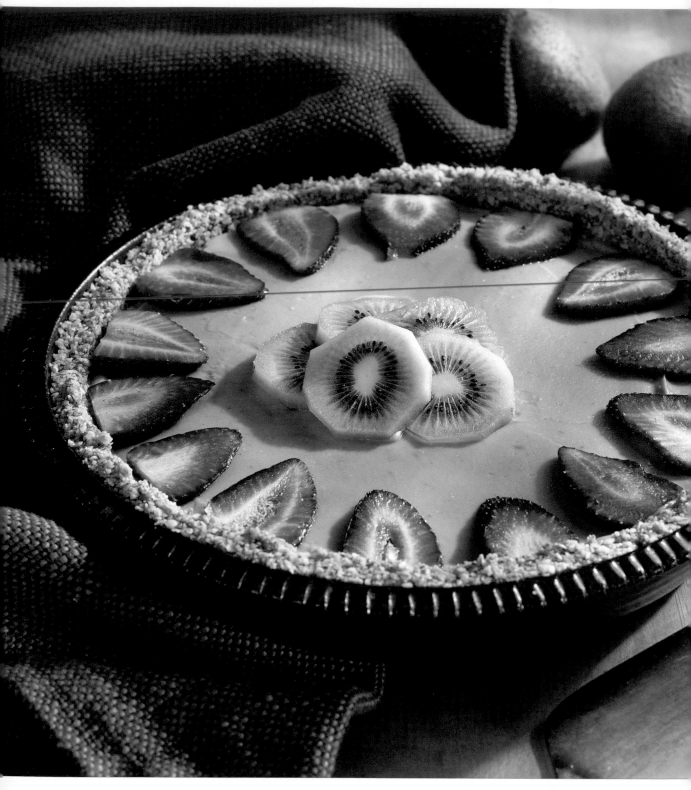

● Loose Stools & Diarrhea ◔ Fiber ◉ Motility and Lubrication ◎ Indigestion ◉ Really Bad Days

Avocado Cream Pie ◎◉

This pie is a full of delicious contradictions. It is smooth yet crunchy, rich yet light, sweet yet sour. It is also packed with nutrients, including healthy fats so portion consciousness is advisable. Gooseberries are said to aid with constipation.

INGREDIENTS

- 4 ripe avocados
- 3 kiwis, peeled and thinly sliced
- 1 cup (220 g) ripe gooseberries or strawberries, halved
- 6 tablespoons (90 ml) lime juice
- 2 tablespoons (28 ml) light agave nectar
- ½ Where-for-Heart-Thou Granola recipe (see page 175)

To make the pie crust, prepare the Where for Heart Thou Granola and puree mixture prior to baking. With your fingers, spread the mixture into a pie pan and refrigerate.

In a food processor, the combine avocado, agave, and lime juice, until creamy. Refrigerate the avocado cream.

To assemble the pie, spread the avocado cream on top of the pie crust. Decorate it with the kiwi and gooseberries, making circles with the kiwi slices overlapping each other on the inside of the pie and one circle of the gooseberries around the outermost edge of the pie. Refrigerate and serve cold.

YIELD: Makes 12 servings.

NUTRITIONAL ANALYSIS

Per Serving: 239 Calories; 18g Fat (3 g saturated fat); 4g Protein; 20g Carbohydrate; 4g Dietary Fiber; 0mg Cholesterol; 9mg Sodium.

"Perfect. Never thought I could have avocado for dessert."

—Claudette

NOTE

You can serve any leftover avocado cream over kiwi and gooseberries in martini glasses.

Halvah°

Raw tahini forms the base of this Middle Eastern favorite. Tahini (made from ground sesame seeds) splits as a protein and fat source that can replace eggs, dairy, and oil in many dishes. See Mediterranean Tofu Scramble (page 44) for a note on who should use sesame for healing.

INGREDIENTS

- Canola oil spray
- 3 cups (430 g) raw sesame seeds
- ¼ cup (60 g) raw sesame tahini
- 1 teaspoon ground ginger
- 1 teaspoon cinnamon
- 1 teaspoon allspice
- ¾ cup (175 ml) agave nectar

Preheat the oven to 350°F (180°C, gas mark 4). Lightly spray a cooking sheet with canola oil spray.

Spread sesame seeds on the prepared sheet. Toast for 3 to 5 minutes, until golden brown. Let cool.

In a food processor, process 2½ cups (360 g) of the sesame seeds (1 cup at a time) with the tahini.

In a mixing bowl, combine the sesame mixture, ginger, cinnamon, allspice, and agave, until well combined. Fold in remaining sesame seeds. Place in a 9-inch (22.5-cm) square pan. Cover with foil and chill overnight. Cut into squares and serve.

YIELD: Makes 20 servings.

NUTRITIONAL ANALYSIS

Per Serving: 178 Calories; 12g Fat (2 g saturated fat); 4g Protein; 16g Carbohydrate; 3g Dietary Fiber; 0mg Cholesterol; 6mg Sodium.

NOTE

If you're concerned about eating whole seeds, process all of the sesame seeds.

"I made this with my mom after school, and I took some to my teacher. She liked it, too."

—Joel, age 9

● Loose Stools & Diarrhea　◉ Fiber　◉ Motility and Lubrication　◎ Indigestion　◎ Really Bad Days

Mochi Mochi Mochi• *choose plain mochi* ⊙ *(diarrhea)*

Mochi are so versatile. They're a welcome stand in for croutons in soup or as hot pockets stuffed with a savory filling or frozen with a sweet surprise inside. They can be made from scratch, but I'd rather spend my cooking time coming up with a stuffing. Plus, today, there are good quality products available. Visit www.grainassance.com if you have trouble finding mochi in your grocery stores. Caution: Frozen mochi are often stuffed with ice cream so ask before you eat or read the label.

INGREDIENTS

- 1 package (12 ounces, or 340 g) mochi
- 1 cup sauce, pudding, spread, or ice cream, such as Hemp-Berry Sauce (page 134), Banana Pudding (page 152), and Spread the Health (page 131)

Preheat the oven to 450°F (230°C, gas mark 8).

Cut the mochi into 2-inch (5-cm) squares. (Smaller squares are difficult to stuff, but they're fine if you're eating the mochi plain or in a soup.) Place the mochi on a baking sheet and bake for 8 to 10 minutes, until the mochi bubble up significantly. Remove from heat and let cool. Use a small spoon to poke a hole at the side of the mochi where the bubbled part meets the flat part. Use a spoon or small funnel to pour the sauce, pudding, spread, or ice cream into the mochi. Serve at room temperature or frozen, depending on stuffing type.

YIELD: Makes 16 mochi.

NUTRITIONAL ANALYSIS
Per Serving: 68 Calories; 1g Fat (0 g saturated fat); 2g Protein; 13g Carbohydrate; trace Dietary Fiber; 0mg Cholesterol; trace Sodium.

"I love these."

—Maggie

Mini Muffins, Big on Taste•• *(diarrhea)*

Kristin's quote says it all. This is delicious treat so good that even the saaviest of kids is likely to confuse these for a chocolate treat.

INGREDIENTS

- ¹/₂ cup (70 g) carob powder
- ³/₄ cup (175 ml) grapeseed oil
- 2 ripe bananas
- ¹/₂ teaspoon sea salt
- 2 teaspoons vanilla extract
- 1 cup (245 g) unsweetened applesauce
- 1 teaspoon cinnamon
- 1 teaspoon xantham gum
- ¹/₄ cup (60 ml) dark agave nectar
- 1 cup (110 g) oat flour
- 1 cup (110 g) all-purpose wheat-free baking mix, such as Arrowhead Mills

Preheat the oven to 350°F (180°C, gas mark 4). Lightly coat a 24-cup mini-muffin sheet with cooking spray or line it with paper muffin cups.

On a baking sheet, spread carob powder into a thin layer. Toast for about 3 to 5 minutes, until the powder hardens and emits a pleasant toasted smell.

Meanwhile, in a food processor, combine the oil, bananas, salt, vanilla, applesauce, cinnamon, xantham, and agave.

In a separate mixing bowl, combine the oat flour and all-purpose baking mix. Add the carob powder once removed from the oven. Combine the mixture from the food processor in with the flour mixture, until no lumps remain. Pour batter into the muffin holders. Bake for 15 to 20 minutes. Let cool and serve or freeze.

YIELD: Makes 24 servings.

NUTRITIONAL ANALYSIS
Per Serving: 157 Calories; 10g Fat (2 g saturated fat); 2g Protein; 17g Carbohydrate; 1g Dietary Fiber; trace Cholesterol; 103mg Sodium.

"Talk about fooling the kids. These could replace brownies, cupcakes, or chocolate muffins!"

—Kristin

NOTE

This recipe was adapted from Bob's Red Mill Carob Applesauce Brownies recipe.

● Loose Stools & Diarrhea ◉ Fiber ◉ Motility and Lubrication ◎ Indigestion ◉ Really Bad Days

Oat Bran–Cherry Mini Muffins°◉

Cherries pop out of these oat bran muffins to add moisture, color, and sweetness. Together with oat bran, the cherries help get the digestive system moving; they are known to detoxify and improve motility of the digestive system, especially the darker ones, which contain more magnesium.

INGREDIENTS

- 1 2/3 cups (185 g) oat flour
- 1 cup (95 g) oat bran
- 2 teaspoons baking powder (ideally aluminum-free)
- 1/2 teaspoon sea salt
- 1/2 teaspoon cinnamon
- 1/4 teaspoon baking soda
- 1/2 cup (120 ml) almond milk
- 1/4 cup (60 ml) light agave nectar
- 1/2 cup unsweetened applesauce
- 18–20 fresh cherries, pitted and finely chopped, or frozen cherries, thawed, and chopped

Preheat the oven to 425°F (220°C, gas mark 7). Coat a mini muffin pan with canola oil spray or line with paper liners.

In a large bowl or food processor, mix the flour, bran, baking powder, salt, cinnamon, and baking soda and stir lightly, just to combine. Set aside.

In another bowl or food processor, combine the milk, agave, and applesauce. Process or mix with a wire whisk until smooth; stir in dry ingredients and combine until a thick but soft dough is formed. Stir in the cherries, gently but thoroughly. Place a soupspoon full of dough into each of the prepared muffin cups. (The dough does not rise, so adjust amount to size of muffin cups.) Bake on the middle rack for 8 to 10 minutes, checking that they are a golden color but not brown. Insert a toothpick or cake tester into center to determine doneness. Cool in pan for 20 minutes and then remove.

YIELD: Makes 18 mini muffins.

NUTRITIONAL ANALYSIS

Per Serving: 177 Calories; 3g Fat (1 g saturated fat); 5g Protein; 3 7g Carbohydrate; 5g Dietary Fiber; 0mg Cholesterol; 283mg Sodium.

"The cherry is like a little sweet surprise."

—Laura

NOTE

These muffins freeze well.

Cashew-Teff Cookies©

Teff may be the tiniest little grain, but it's quite big on taste and nutrient content. It's rich in minerals. Split here with rice flour to soften teff's typical grittiness, teff brings an "Is this chocolate?" flavor to these cookies.

INGREDIENTS

- Canola oil spray
- $^3/_4$ cup (135 g) teff
- $^3/_4$ cup (85 g) sweet rice flour
- $^1/_2$ teaspoon salt
- $^1/_3$ cup (75 ml) dark agave nectar
- $^1/_4$ cup (60 ml) canola oil
- 1 teaspoon vanilla
- $^1/_2$ cup (120 g) creamy cashew butter
- 1 egg or 1/4 cup unsweetened applesauce

Preheat the oven 350ºF (180°C, gas mark 4). Lightly coat a cookie sheet with canola oil spray.

In a food processor, blend the dry ingredients to make a flour. Blend in the wet ingredients. Pinch off little balls and place them on the prepared cookie sheet, pressing each cookie flat with the back of a fork. Bake for 12 to 15 minutes; remove from the oven, and cool on racks.

YIELD: Makes 30 cookies.

NUTRITIONAL ANALYSIS
Per Serving: 69 Calories; 4g Fat (1 g saturated fat); 1g Protein; 7g Carbohydrate; trace Dietary Fiber; 6mg Cholesterol; 38mg Sodium.

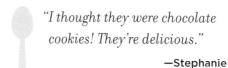

"I thought they were chocolate cookies! They're delicious."

—Stephanie

● Loose Stools & Diarrhea   ◐ Fiber   ◉ Motility and Lubrication   ◎ Indigestion   ◉ Really Bad Days

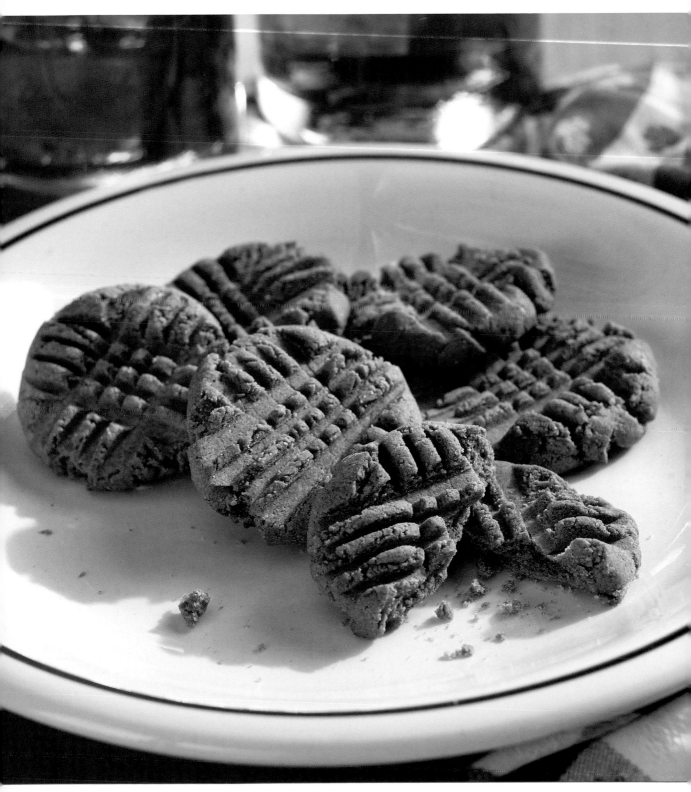

Coco-nana-nut Cookies°⊙

In this recipe several ingredients complement each other for a moist, mildly sweet cookie or bar. The combination also suits IBS sufferers quite nicely as the nutrients here help add bulk, improve motility, and help maintain a supportive environment for good bacteria.

INGREDIENTS

- 3 ripe bananas, mashed
- 1 teaspoon vanilla extract
- ¼ cup (60 g) unsweetened applesauce
- ¼ cup (60 ml) dark agave nectar
- ½ cup (120 ml) canola oil
- 1 tablespoon (14 ml) coconut milk
- 1 teaspoon baking soda
- 1 cup (110 g) oat flour
- 1 teaspoon cinnamon
- 1 cup (100 g) rolled oats
- 1 cup (80 g) shredded coconut

Preheat the oven to 350°F (180°C, gas mark 4). Lightly coat a cookie sheet with cooking spray.

In a food processor, blend the bananas, vanilla, applesauce, agave, oil, and coconut milk. Once combined, add in the baking soda, flour, and cinnamon. Fold in oats and coconut by hand. Using two teaspoons, scoop dough onto the prepared cookie sheet. Bake for 18 to 20 minutes.

YIELD: Makes 30 cookies.

NUTRITIONAL ANALYSIS

Per Serving: 94 Calories; 5g Fat (1 g saturated fat); 2g Protein; 11g Carbohydrate; 1g Dietary Fiber; 0mg Cholesterol; 43mg Sodium.

"This is our household's new favorite."

—Claire and Chris

 Loose Stools & Diarrhea ● Fiber ◉ Motility and Lubrication ◎ Indigestion 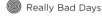 Really Bad Days

Grab 'n Go Granola Bars °◉

A truly satisfying snack or meal, you can feel good about eating this granola bar—as good as it will make you feel. The recipe can be made raw as a tasty vehicle for prebiotic powder (see resource section on page 180), which helps to enable a hospitable environment for the good guys (good bacteria).

INGREDIENTS

- 1¹/₂ cups (150 g) rolled oats
- ³/₄ cup (190 g) favorite nut butter, such as almond
- ¹/₂ cup (50 g) chopped mixed nuts
- 1 tablespoon (14 ml) plus 1 teaspoon dark agave nectar
- ¹/₄ cup (40 g) buckwheat groats
- ¹/₄ cup (40 g) oat groats
- ¹/₄ cup (56 g) Goji berries
- 1 teaspoon vanilla extract
- ¹/₄ cup (15 g) prebiotic powder (only use if making raw recipe)
- ¹/₄ cup (60 g) hemp seeds
- 2 tablespoons (30 g) black sesame seeds
- ¹/₂ cup crystallized ginger
- ¹/₂ cup (20 g) unsweetened, shredded coconut

If you intend to bake the bars, preheat the oven to 350°F (180°C, gas mark 4). Lightly coat a 9-inch (22.5-cm) square baking dish with cooking spray.

In a food processor, process the nut butter, vanilla, and prebiotic powder (only use prebiotic powder if making raw recipe). Add in nuts, ginger, and groats and pulse to combine. (Do not over process, the mixture should be chunky.)

In a large mixing bowl, place the oats, seeds, berries, and coconut. Fold in the nut mixture and combine well. Add agave to taste. Spread the mixture into the prepared baking dish, using the back of a spatula. If eating raw, let sit for a few minutes, cut, and serve. Otherwise bake for 7 to 10 minutes. Let cool before cutting into bars.

YIELD: Makes approximately 25 1" square bars.

NUTRITIONAL ANALYSIS
Per Serving: 134 Calories; 8g Fat (1 g saturated fat); 4g Protein; 12g Carbohydrate; 2g Dietary Fiber; 0mg Cholesterol; 4mg Sodium.

"Great. Just as good as the unhealthy stuff."

—Mike

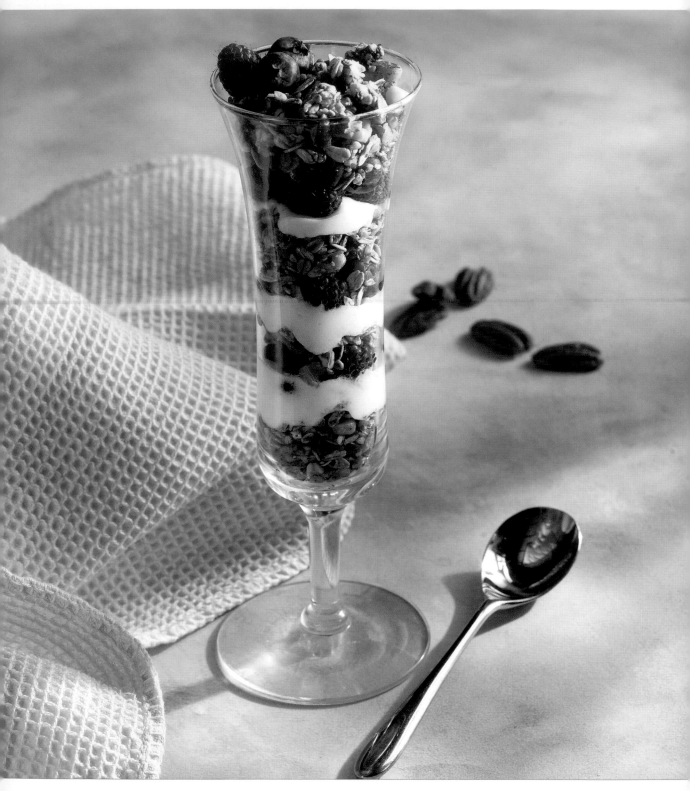

● Loose Stools & Diarrhea ◐ Fiber ◉ Motility and Lubrication ◎ Indigestion ◉ Really Bad Days

Where-for-Heart-Thou Granola°◉

Full of taste and texture and overflowing with nutrient power, your heart will feel good whether eating this granola or preparing it for someone you love. What's more, each of the ingredients selected brings an impressive resume for healthy digestion.

INGREDIENTS

- 1¹/₂ cups (150 g) rolled oats
- 1 cup (100 g) finely chopped assorted raw, unsalted nuts, such as pistachios, pine nuts, almonds, and walnuts
- 1 tablespoon (14 ml) plus 1 teaspoon dark agave nectar
- ¹/₄ cup (40 g) buckwheat groats
- 1 teaspoon vanilla extract
- 1 teaspoon cinnamon
- 3 teaspoons ground flaxseeds
- 2 tablespoons (30 g) hemp seeds
- ¹/₃ cup (75 ml) grapeseed oil

Preheat the oven to 350°F (180°C, gas mark 4). Lightly coat a cookie sheet with cooking spray.

In a mixing bowl, combine all ingredients well and place on the prepared cookie sheet. Bake for about 10 minutes, stirring occasionally, until golden brown. Let cool.

YIELD: Makes 10 servings.

NUTRITIONAL ANALYSIS

Per Serving: 244 Calories, 18g Fat (2 g saturated fat), 8g Protein, 18g Carbohydrate; 4g Dietary Fiber; 0mg Cholesterol; 3mg Sodium.

"This granola is totally unique and amazing. What is in it?"

—Vanessa

NOTE

The nuts are best if frozen.

Berry-Rice Pudding ●◎

Here traditional rice pudding, which is often deemed too bland, gets a full makeover. Ingredients like hemp seeds, ginger, berries, and even Goji berries, decorate with flavor, color, and texture. Goji berries are sold dried, but they moisten up when cooked into the pudding. Loaded with mineral and vitamins, the Goji berry comes to us from Tibet.

INGREDIENTS

- 1 cup (235 ml) unsweetened rice milk
- 1 cup (200 g) cooked brown rice
- $1/2$ cup (65 g) mixed berries, such as raspberries, blackberries, and blueberries
- 2 tablespoons (56 g) Goji berries
- 2 teaspoons ground ginger
- 3 teaspoons hemp seeds (optional)

In a saucepan, bring all ingredients to a boil. Reduce the heat to low and simmer for about 20 minutes, stirring occasionally. (The cooking time depends on the desired consistency.)

YIELD: Makes 4 servings.

NUTRITIONAL ANALYSIS
Per Serving: 102 Calories; 2g Fat (trace saturated fat); 3g Protein; 18g Carbohydrate; 2g Dietary Fiber; 0mg Cholesterol; 3mg Sodium.

"This hits the spot in the morning."
—Sally

● Loose Stools & Diarrhea   ◐ Fiber   ◉ Motility and Lubrication   ◎ Indigestion   ◎ Really Bad Days

Sample Menus

Quantity is one serving unless otherwise noted.

Day One

DAY 1	MEAL 1	MEAL 2	MEAL 3	SNACK 1	SNACK 2
CONSTIPATION —FIBER	QuintesSensual Quinoa (**PAGE 40**)	Fennel–White Bean Soup (**PAGE 82**) and Veggie Chips (**PAGE 122**)	Turkey Meatballs (**PAGE 64**) and Brightly Sautéed Greens (**PAGE 117**)	Apple or pear	Spinach Balls (2–3) (**PAGE 86**)
CONSTIPATION —MOTILITY AND LUBRICATION	Grapefruit-Adzuki Salad (**PAGE 111**)	Spinach-Artichoke Dip (**PAGE 136**) and Oat Crackers (**PAGE 124**)	3 S Scramble (**PAGE 52**)	Halvah (**PAGE 166**)	Baked Apples (**PAGE 150**)
REALLY BAD DAY— CONSTIPATION	Stewed Figs (**PAGE 160**) and hemp seeds	A Hummus the Whole Body Will Love (**PAGE 139**) and Veggie Chips (**PAGE 122**)	Omega-3 Lasagna (**PAGE 55**)	Iced Revelation (**PAGE 147**) or Letting-Go Latte (**PAGE 143**)	Nobody's Rhubarb Fool (**PAGE 151**)
LOOSE STOOLS /DIARRHEA	Everything-but-the-Kitchen-Sink Hash (**PAGE 49**)	Nixed the Noodles for Spaghetti Pad Thai (**PAGE 53**)	Turkey Wraps (**PAGE 66**) made with Timeless Tapenade (**PAGE 129**)	Iced Berry Sangri-Tea (**PAGE 145**)	Mochi Mochi Mochi (**PAGE 167**) stuffed with Banana Pudding (**PAGE 152**)
REALLY BAD DAY— DIARRHEA	Calming Congee (**PAGE 39**) or Millet Marvel Congee (**PAGE 39**)	Scrambled egg whites and Banana Pudding (**PAGE 152**)	Gut Healer (**PAGE 146**)	Artisan Applesauce (**PAGE 132**)	"They'll All Root for This" Vegetable Medley (**PAGE 121**)
GAS/BLOATING /INDIGESTION	Millet Marvel Congee (**PAGE 39**)	SAAG-sational (**PAGE 45**) and Fish 'n Chips, minus the chips (**PAGE 59**)	Papaya Soup (**PAGE 79**) and "Jerk" Turkey Burgers (**PAGE 65**)	Zucchini Boats (**PAGE 95**) and No Más Gas Guacamole (**PAGE 137**)	Peppermint Sooth-E (**PAGE 143**)

Day Two

DAY 2	MEAL 1	MEAL 2	MEAL 3	SNACK 1	SNACK 2
CONSTIPATION —FIBER	Heart 'n Colon Porridge (PAGE 48)	Dairy-Free, Oh-So-Tasty Fish Chowder (PAGE 82) and Veggie Chips (PAGE 124)	Buffalo Chili (PAGE 74) or Pork-Tendered for Better Digestion (PAGE 77)	Berries (1 cup)	Zucchini Boats (PAGE 95) and Omega-3 Pesto (PAGE 127)
CONSTIPATION —MOTILITY AND LUBRICATION	Oat Bran—Cherry Mini Muffins (PAGE 103)	Chicken Wrappers (PAGE 100) and Sweet 'n Crispy Seaweed Salad (PAGE 110)	Stir-Fried Scallops and Sweet Potatoes (PAGE 56)	Zucchini Boats (PAGE 95) and Gingerly Twisted Gomasio Sauce (PAGE 133)	Devilish Eggs (PAGE 90) and Prune-Ginger Chutney (PAGE 128)
REALLY BAD DAY— CONSTIPATION	Sesame-Vegetable Pâté (PAGE 88)	Fig-Chicken Curry (PAGE 69)	Kasha-Stuffed Tomatoes (PAGE 97)	Peach Soup (PAGE 78)	Brightly Sautéed Greens (PAGE 117)
LOOSE STOOLS / DIARRHEA	Gnocchi Sweet Gnocchi (PAGE 43)	Fish 'n Chips (PAGE 59)	Mary's Risotto Salad (PAGE 106)	Baked Apples (PAGE 150)	ProHydrator (PAGE 139)
REALLY BAD DAY— DIARRHEA	Spooner's Chestnut Soup (PAGE 81)	Mini-Muffins, Big on Taste (PAGE 168)	Chicken-Mushroom Risotto (PAGE 72)	Iced Berry Sangri-Tea (PAGE 145)	Gut Healer (PAGE 146)
GAS/BLOATING /INDIGESTION	Peppermint Sooth-E (PAGE 143)	Lime Fish Kebabs (PAGE 54) and Suitable Slaw (PAGE 109)	Turkey Wraps (PAGE 66), with No Más Gas Guacamole (PAGE 137)	Ginger-AID (PAGE 146)	Digestif-ly Pleasing Poached Pears (PAGE 153)

Day Three

DAY 3	MEAL 1	MEAL 2	MEAL 3	SNACK 1	SNACK 2
CONSTIPATION —FIBER ◉	Grab 'n Go Granola Bars (PAGE 174)	Salmon-Celeriac Salad (PAGE 93) and Zucchini Boats (PAGE 95)	Lentil-Amaranth Pancakes (PAGE 120) and Prune-Ginger Chutney (PAGE 128) and SAAG-sational (PAGE 45)	Spinach Balls (2-3) (PAGE 86)	Apple or pear
CONSTIPATION —MOTILITY AND LUBRICATION ◉	Turkey slices and Sweet-Tart Baked Gram Pistachio Pear Salad (PAGE 105)	Sesame-Ginger Fish and Greens (PAGE 61) and Kristin's Mashed "I Can't Believe It's Not Potato" Cauliflower (PAGE 119)	I Ieart 'n Colon Porridge (PAGE 46)	Iced Revelation (PAGE 147)	Devilish Eggs (PAGE 90) and Tri-Color Salsa (PAGE 126)
REALLY BAD DAY— CONSTIPATION ◎	Baked Apples (PAGE 150)	Chicken Bouillabaisse (PAGE 67)	Deeply Greens au Gratin, with optional turkey or chicken breast (PAGE 118)	Truly *Naturally* Decaffeinated Tea (PAGE 142) and Oat Crackers (PAGE 124)	Divine Berry Crisp (PAGE 148)
LOOSE STOOLS / DIARRHEA ●	Berry-Rice Pudding (PAGE 175)	Root Vegetable– Chicken–Apple Sausage Stew (PAGE 68) or Raspberry Chicken (PAGE 73)	Scrambled egg whites and Buck-the-Wheat Tortillas (PAGE 119)	Artisan Applesauce (PAGE 132)	Iced Berry Sangri-Tea (PAGE 145)
REALLY BAD DAY— DIARRHEA ◎	Calming Congee (PAGE 39) or Millet Marvel Congee (PAGE 39)	Fish 'n Chips (PAGE 59)	Pumpkin Punch (PAGE 82)	Herbal tea	ProHydrator (PAGE 139)
GAS/BLOATING /INDIGESTION ◎	Gut Healer (PAGE 146)	Turkey Wraps (PAGE 66), with Pineapple Chutney (PAGE 85)	Over-the-Moon Mini Crab Cakes (PAGE 98) and On-a-Greens-Kick Soup (PAGE 85)	Veggie Chips (PAGE 122)	Ginger-AID (PAGE 146) or Peppermint Sooth-E (PAGE 143)

Resources

The following provides resources that will further help you on your healing path. In some instances either a phone number or Web site appears as the preferred contact option. Note: A special thanks to Whole Foods markets for continuing to make quality food products (like those listed below) available.

FOOD COMPANIES

Nuts, seeds, beans, and granola

Lydia's Organics
www.lydiasorganics.com
415-258-9678

Bear Naked granola
www.bearnakedgranola.com

Savory Suns (seeds)
805-594-1924

Living Harvest
(hemp seeds / hemp protein powder)
www.livingharvest.com
888-690-3958

Diamond of California
www.diamondnuts.com
209-467-6000

Barleans Forti Flax
www.barleans.com
800-445-3529

Eden Foods Inc.
www.edenfoods.com
888-441-3336

nSpired Natural Foods
www.nspiredfoods.com
510-346-3860

Sun Organic Farm
(chia seeds)
www.sunorganic.com
888-269-9888

Oils, sauces, and spreads

Spectrum Organics Products
www.spectrumorganics.com
La Tourangelle
www.latourangelle.com
(Williams Sonoma)

Bragg's
www.bragg.com
800-446-1990

Living Harvest
(hemp oil)
www.livingharvest.com
888-690-3958

Agave Nectar
www.sweetcactusfarms.com
310-837-7554

Thai Kitchen
www.thaikitchen.com
800-967-THAI

Ginger People
www.gingerpeople.com
800-551-5284

Muir Glen Organic
www.cfarm.com
800-624-4123

Produce

Earthbound Farms
www.ebfarms.com
800-690-3200

Sambazon (acai)
www.sambazon.com
877-736-2296

Animal Proteins:

Applegate Farms
www.applegatefarms.com
866-587-5858

Eggology Inc.
www.eggology.com
818-610-2222

Breads, tortillas, flours, etc.

French Meadow bakery
www.frenchmeadow.com
877 NO YEAST

Nairn's
www.nairns-oatcakes.com

Arrowhead Mills
www.arrowheadmills.com
800-434-4246

Bob's Red Mills
www.bobsredmill.com
800-349-2173

Jay Robb
egg white protein powder
www.jayrobb.com

Beverages

In pursuit of tea
www.inpursuitoftea.com
860-672-4768

O.N.E.
coconut water
www.onenaturalexperience.com;
Whole Foods

Triple Leaf Tea
www.tripleleaf-tea.com
800-552-7448

Yogi Tea
www.yogitea.com
800-YOGITEA

Teeccino Caffe, Inc.
www.teeccino.com
800-498-3434

Ginger People
www.gingerpeople.com
800-551-5284

Emergen-C
www.alacer.com
800-854-0249

Supplement companies

(These are those that I commonly recommend; there are many other good quality products available, discuss your options with a qualified healthcare practitioner.)

Metagenics
www.metagenics.com
800-692-9400

Designs for Health
www.designsforhealth.com
800-847-8302

Ortho Molecular Products
www.orthomolecularproducts.com
800-332-2351

Nordic Naturals
www.nordicnaturals.com
800.662.2544 x1

New Chapter
www.newchapter.info
800-543-7279

Natural Calm
www.naturalclam.net
(800) 446-7462

Yerba Prima
www.yerba.com
800-488-4339

Flora Stor
www.florastor.com

Gaia herbs
www.gaiaherbs.com

WEIL
www.drweil.com

References

1. Sandler RS, Everhart JE, Donowitz M et al. The burden of selected digestive diseases in the United States. *Gastroenterology* 2002;122:1500-1511.

2. Gralneck IM, Hays RD, Kilbourne A, et al. The impact of irritable bowel syndrome on health-related quality of life. *Gastroenterology* 2000;119:654-660.

3. Hahn BA, Kirchdoerfer LJ, Fullerton S, et al. Patient-perceived severity of irritable bowel syndrome in relation to symptoms, health resource utilization, and quality of life. *Alimentary Pharmacology and Therapeutics* 1997;11:553-559.

4. Drossman DA, Li Z, Andruzzi E, et al. U.S. householder survey of functional gastrointestinal disorders. Prevalence, sociodemography, and health impact. *Digestive Diseases Sciences* 1993;38:1569-1580.

5. Frank L, Kleinman L, Rentz A, et al. Health related quality of life associated with irritable bowel syndrome: comparison with other chronic issues. *Clinical Therapeutics* 2002;24:675-689.

6. Whitehead WE, Holtkotter B, Enck P, et al. Tolerance for rectosigmoid distention in irritable bowel syndrome. *Gastroenterology* 1990;98:1187-1192.

7. Silverman DH, Munakata JA, Ennes H, et al. Regional cerebral activity in normal and pathological perception of visceral pain. *Gastroenterology* 1997;112:64-72.

8. Lawal A, Kern M, Sidhu H, et al. Novel evidence for hypersensitivity of visceral sensory neural circuitry in irritable bowel syndrome patients. *Gastroenterology* 2006;130:26-33.

9. Bueno L, Fioramonti J, Delvaux M, et al. Mediators and pharmacology of visceral sensitivity: from basic to clinical investigations. *Gastroenterology* 1997;112:1714-1743.

10. Goyal RK, Hirano I. The enteric nervous system. *New England Journal of Medicine* 1996;334:1106-1115.

11. Tillisch K, Chang L. Diagnosis and treatment of irritable bowel syndrome: State of the art. *Current Gastroenterology Reports* 2005;7(4):249-256.

12. Thompson WG, Heaton KW, Smyth GT, et al. Irritable bowel syndrome in general practice: prevalence, characteristics, and referral. *Gut* 2000 46(1):78-82.

13. Tack J, Broekaert D, Fischler B, et al. A controlled cross-over study of the selective serotonin reuptake inhibitor citalopram in irritable bowel syndrome. *Gut* 2006 55(8):1096-1103.

14. Vahedi H, Merat S, Rashidioon A, et al. The effect of fluoxetine in patients with pain and constipation-predominant irritable bowel syndrome: a double-blind randomized-controlled study. *Alimentary Pharmacology and Therapeutics* 2005;22(5):381-385.

15. Reilly MC, Bargout V, McBurney CR, et al. Effect of tegaserod on work and daily activity in irritable bowel syndrome with constipation. *Alimentary Pharmacology and Therapeutics* 2005;22(5):373-80.

16. O'Mahony L, Mccarthy J, Kelly P, et al. Lactobacillus and Bifidobacterium in irritable bowel syndrome: symptom responses and relationship to cytokine profiles. *Gastroenterology* 2005;128:541-551.

Common Eating Traps

Here are a few final notes to think about.

The Appetite versus Hunger Trap

Hunger and appetite are not synonyms; hunger is the physiologic need for food, whereas appetite speaks to desire for food triggered by the senses or emotions. It is a common trap to confuse the two and eat in an effort to satisfy appetite beyond or in the absence of hunger. Identifying whether hunger or appetite as the trigger for your food need helps you to eat for optimal digestion.

The Thirst versus Hunger Trap

Being thirsty can mimic being hungry. Furthermore, dehydration is implicated in digestive problems (i.e., constipation) and headaches, which can trigger poor quality food choices. Ask yourself, are you thirsty or hungry? Did you recently eat? Was your meal salty? Are you suffering from diarrhea? Did you just workout? When did you last drink water or a water-based beverage? Try drinking some water before making a food choice. At best, you quench your thirst. At worst, you're still hungry and can rule out thirst as a cause.

The Too-Hungry-to-Think Trap

Letting oneself get too hungry by skipping meals, waiting too long, or eating too little typically sets one up for failure. When too hungry, we succumb to common food traps—eating something just because it's around, eating what appeals to our senses (not what's right for our system), eating too quickly, and overeating, which often trigger gastrointestinal distress.

The Eating-Out Trap

Eating out exposes you to many potential traps. When it comes to eating out, your best defense is offense—prepare. Here are some things to keep in mind:

REDUCE THE RISK OF BEING TOO HUNGRY TO THINK.

- SNACK HEALTHFULLY. Bring snacks with you (ideally) or purchase a snack if it might be more than 3 to 4 hours between eating occasions. This is also a great idea if you are not sure about the quality of food that will be available for your next meal.

- **DON'T SKIP OR SKIMP ON DAYTIME MEALS.** I call it *backloading* when a client eats too little (in an effort to be good or because the day is too crazy) during the day and then over-consumes at night. Skipping meals or eating too little can set you up for failure.

REDUCE TEMPTATION.

- Ask the waitperson to skip the bread or fries or other temptation when ordering.
- Don't set yourself up for failure. It's hard to sit in an ice cream shop and not eat ice cream, or not drink coffee in a coffee shop, or not eat candy at a candy store. You get my drift. If you have to go somewhere that might not have anything for you, bring yourself a treat.

REDUCE FRUSTRATION.

- Whenever possible, choose an eating establishment that you know well. Sometimes the choice is not yours but you can request a certain type of cuisine. Otherwise, check out the menu for a new place (call or look online).
- Be "a Sally," as in Meg Ryan's character from *When Harry Met Sally*. Order meals the way you like them, even if others poke fun at you for being particular. Don't forget to smile and be patient when ordering; being pleasant helps the wait staff know you appreciate their efforts to get you the meal you want.

INCREASE SUCCESS.

- Knowledge is power. Learn how to order (what are the right questions), about food and food preparations; doing your best when dining out requires making an effort to be an informed patron and conscious eater. Remember that you are paying for both your food and your experience. If you don't know what a food is or how it's prepared, ask. A good chef and wait staff should appreciate your desire to educate yourself about their preparations.
- Always bring a gift for your guest—and yourself. Call ahead and offer to bring a part of the meal or an appetizer; make it something that you know you enjoy and tolerate well. You'll be less stressed for the get together and your host will undoubtedly appreciate your effort.

- Modify the adventure. While you don't have to go with the same food all the time, you may want to rely on some staples. This holds especially true for times when you are dealing with a particularly sensitive digestive system or are already nervous in your dining situation (such as an important business dinner may not be the time to experiment). Think small and simple. Rarely will one bite of food trigger symptoms.

LEARN THE COMMON DINING OUT TRAPS.

- **DAIRY.** Even if you're not avoiding dairy entirely, you should be aware that dairy is often used in cooking, even where you might not suspect it, as well as in larger quantities. Ask before you order, but be especially aware of soups (cream bases), sauces, sautéed foods, breads, baked goods, desserts, and shakes or smoothies.

- **WHEAT FLOUR.** Most breads, pizza crusts, baked goods, and crackers contain wheat flour. Some artisan breads may use flours from other grains, but still typically include a significant amount of wheat flour. Also, some healthier soup recipes use wheat flour as part of their stock.

- **FROZEN YOGURT SHOPS.** Few people (even non-IBS sufferers) survive frozen yogurt without increased flatulence and bloating. While I recommend avoiding, if you choose to indulge, keep it to a small amount. Also, it appears to be more bothersome to a truly empty stomach.

- **FOOD SAFETY.** How long is the food kept out? Observe others around you. Are they eating from the bar directly, sneezing, or coughing near the food? Do the vegetables appear to be swimming in grease or are your greens looking a bit brown? Special attention should be paid to food sitting out at salad bars or other buffet style restaurants, as well as food sold at airports and malls.

- **HEALTH FOOD.** Some of the healthiest cuisines, even "health foods," can be harmful to the digestive system, and actually unhealthy overall. Steer clear of fast food versions of cuisines from around the world because they often bare little resemblance to the real thing. Mystery sauces, excessively greasy food, extremely large portions, and mono-color meals should be passed in favor of trying an authentic dish at home or at a restaurant of well-known quality.

PREPARE A DEFENSE BECAUSE SOMETIMES EVEN THE BEST OFFENSE DOESN'T WORK.

- Lessen the blow. Smaller portions or less frequent consumption of foods or beverages less good for you also helps to reduce long-term irritation.

- An incorrect choice today begets a correct one tomorrow. Learn from mistakes.

The Breakfast Traps

Some people *are* morning people, and some people are *not*. Likewise, some stomachs are early risers and others struggle with the break of day. Because how you feel in the morning significantly impacts the rest of your day, getting in tune with what works for you in the morning makes good sense. Some common breakfast blunders and bright ideas follow below.

SKIPPING. Breakfast is the most important meal of the day. You are breaking a fast. In terms of metabolism and weight management, breakfast gets your body in the using, not storing mode. Additionally, in terms of optimizing digestion, breakfast, specifically the right breakfast for you, can ease your system into a successful day.

COFFEE FIRST, OR ONLY. If you choose to drink coffee, choose to not drink it on an empty stomach. Take an empty stomach and pour some coffee in—a known gastric acid stimulant—and voila, GI disaster. Eating or drinking a little something before or with your coffee can help lessen the sting.

SAVOR THE MORNING. Savory breakfasts can start your day just right. There's no such thing as a breakfast food. If herb-roasted root vegetables and some fish sound good for breakfast, enjoy this satisfying, healthy, and digestively good food for you start to the day.

DRINKING VERSUS EATING BREAKFAST. Smoothies can be a delicious, nutrient-dense, and convenient breakfast. However, for many people, drinking breakfast does not satisfy as much as a chewing a meal would. Discover what works for you. If you do choose a smoothie, drink slowly, watch your portion, and perhaps include some fiber (like ground flaxseeds or oat or rice bran). If a smoothie is not as filling as another breakfast, prepare by bringing a snack with you for the mid-morning.

THE MORNING FIBER OVER-LOAD. Yes, fiber is a critical part of a healthy nutrition plan. Most people will benefit from increasing the amount of fiber they consume. However, too much fiber at any one time, especially in the morning, can trigger the very symptoms you're working to avoid. Spread fiber intake throughout the day, and your system will likely respond better. Additionally, make sure to hydrate adequately to digest the fiber.

YOUR FIBER LOAD. While cereal or oatmeal with ground flaxseeds, berries, and nuts makes for a wonderful breakfast for some, for others it's a recipe for GI disaster. Maybe you'd do better with egg whites and veggies for breakfast or congee or sardines on toast. Discover your fiber load, what works for your body, and increase the amount as your system tolerates.

GIVE YOUR COLON (AND THE REST OF YOU) A GOOD STRETCH. Stretches, such as chair twists and bending from the waist help waken up your body, including your digestive system. Take a yoga or stretch class, rent a video, find a qualified instructor or grab a book to learn about these and other movements to help get you and your system moving each morning.

How to Trick the Traps

The trick to overcoming the traps is preparation. How do we prepare? We plan. I often take my clients through scenarios to help identify options for different situations. The key here is to develop several options to increase the potential for a single successful result. Sure you can plan to bring food to work, but what option exists if your morning was hectic and you forget it or you didn't have anything at home to bring? Scenario planning goes through each of these possibilities, to develop potential solutions, so that ultimately you have an option, even two, for most situations.

Help for Really Bad Days

IBS sufferers know there are good days, not-so good days, and really bad days. Recognizing there may be really bad days, especially in the beginning, certain recipes, strategies, and lifestyle recommendations may help lessen their intensity and duration. In this book, a purple circle denotes recipes best suited to help on these exceptionally distressful days.

What's the goal for a really bad day? It's simple?to get through it. Here are a few thoughts, besides the recipes, that may help.

GET SLEEP. Whether its diarrhea, constipation, excessive gas and bloating, or cramps, you're more than likely worn out from dealing with your symptoms. If at all possible, sneak in a nap and plan for as early a night as feasible. After all, the best way to get through a really bad day is to end it.

RELY ON ONE REMEDY AND ONE REMEDY ALONE. Maybe you already know one that works for you. If not, after reading about some of the options (hopefully you've been able to do this in advance and have an option at home) pick one to try and see if it helps. A really bad day is not the day to try several new remedies at once.

POSTPONE THE UNNECESSARY. Whatever is on your to-do list will get one better and less painfully to tomorrow than if you push yourself on a really bad day. Finish the necessities and then call it a day. One day off does not make you lazy or irresponsible.

CONTEMPLATE OR DOCUMENT, BUT DON'T OVERANALYZE, THE TRIGGER. Some patients come in the day(s) after a really bad day really stressed out because they are still trying to figure out what upset their system. As valuable as the information may be, the relentless stress of identifying a cause may prolong the bad of a really bad day. On a really bad day, take some notes; wait for a better day to evaluate patterns in your food-symptom journal or discuss with your healthcare practitioner.

GET SOME FORM OF ACTIVITY. Remember that relaxation efforts count and may be the perfect anecdote to a really bad day. The goal is to up your body, as opposed to giving into any contraction or tightness you may feel. Swimming, massage, or a walk are just a few examples of activities that may keep your body (and mind) open to the possibility of feeling better tomorrow.

Index

Acknowledgments

Here, too, it is the ingredients that enable a successful recipe—mine—for happiness and health.

The *quality* basics—the principles—are my family. I literally couldn't have completed this project without my mother's help; thanks for putting you true art aside to help enable mine. Now get thee back to the studio! Dad, you were the first to teach me about mise en place, I dedicate that section to you. My brothers, my sisters (in-law and in-my-good-fortune), and my "so advanced" nephew, you each show me different flavors and textures and how they combine to delicious perfection. And to Grandma, you are and will always be my favorite enabler.

The supporting cast—my friends—I am thankful for each of you. Whether my ideas are recipes for success or disaster, you honor me with a laugh, a smile, an ear, and a hug. Furthermore, you allow me to further my knowledge with humorous but real discussions of bowel problems, remedies, and results, which is above and beyond the call of duty but so appreciated.

The extras—an incredible assortment of colleagues, patients, instructors, and practitioners who teach with words and example. Thanks to Dr. Mitchell Spirt, Dr. Soram Khalsa, Dr. Bijan Pourat, Dr. Susan Mandel, Dr. Tannenbaum, Dr. Eitches, Dr. Baum, Dr. Verma, Drs. Mao, Tan, and Dao, David Fabrizio, and Dr. Ed Phillips for your ongoing support. Thank you to Bill, Elise, Ron, Kristin, Patsy, Marilyn, Rach, Laurie and Lynn, Steve, Jill, Karen, Judy, and so many more.

The finales—My Top TEN, especially nutrient L—were taught to me by my family and without it, neither my career nor this book would have come to fruition. The rest include Iyengar yoga, massages, Shel Silverstein, swimming pools and swing sets, California, fresh flowers, and visionaries such as Dr. Andrew Weil and Dr. Jeffrey Bland.

About the Author

Ashley Koff is a registered dietitian trained in all aspects of nutritional counseling. Educated at Duke and New York Universities, Ashley Koff, R.D., trained in clinical dietetics at Los Angeles and USC County Hospital. She founded the Healthxchange— a nutrition counseling and consulting company—in 2002. Currently, she sees patients privately and is on staff at Cedars-Sinai Medical Center in Los Angeles, California, where she lives.

Ashley Koff, R.D., has appeared as a health expert on CNN and on television shows, including *Celebrity Fit Club 3*, *The Ultimate Goal*, and *Brunch*. She is a sought-after public speaker for both healthcare professionals and the general public— both children and adults. She describes her mission as "to help people realize their personal health goals—one healthXchange at a time."